Springer Series on Child and Family Studies

Series Editor

Nirbhay N. Singh, Medical College of Georgia, Augusta University, Augusta, USA

The Springer Series on Child and Family Studies addresses fundamental psychological, educational, social, and related issues within the context of child and family research. Volumes published in this series examine clinical topics with an additional focus on epidemiological, developmental, and life span issues. Leading scholars explore such factors as race and immigration, parenting, and the effects of war and violence on military families and unite a vast literature into a comprehensive series of related research volumes.

Laura K. Taylor · Jessica Surdey · Seaneen Sloan
Editors

Growing Up in Digital Europe

GUIDE's Cross-National Longitudinal Research on Child Wellbeing

Springer

Editors
Laura K. Taylor
School of Psychology
University College Dublin
Dublin, Ireland

Jessica Surdey
School of Education
University College Dublin
Dublin, Ireland

Seaneen Sloan
School of Education
University College Dublin
Dublin, Ireland

ISSN 2570-0421 ISSN 2570-043X (electronic)
Springer Series on Child and Family Studies
ISBN 978-3-032-30591-6 ISBN 978-3-032-30592-3 (eBook)
https://doi.org/10.1007/978-3-032-30592-3

This work was supported by The European Education and Culture Executive Agency.

This Springer imprint is published by the registered company Springer Nature Switzerland AG
The registered company address is: Gewerbestrasse 11, 6330 Cham, Switzerland

Foreword

Over the past two decades, there have been significant advances in the availability and quality of population data across the world. Scientists and policymakers are increasingly using these data to inform social policies and identify interventions with positive societal benefits. The most useful data for these purposes comes from individuals, taking into account their family situation, and measured over time.

Some countries have a deep history of collecting and using such high-quality evidence. Across Europe, collective efforts to pool knowledge also have taken root. For example, the Survey of Health Aging and Retirement in Europe (SHARE) is a longitudinal study of 50+ year olds surveyed regularly across 28 member countries. Other examples of cross-national, representative surveys exist and are regularly used to provide evidence for science and policy. There has until now, however, been an important gap in the data landscape; that is where the GUIDE Book steps in.

Growing Up in Digital Europe (GUIDE), which is detailed in this book, is a groundbreaking project which, for the first time, collects harmonized data about children as they grow up. Credit must be given to the European Commission, who addressed this lacuna in 2013 when they funded a study on the feasibility and desirability of such a project. Over ten years later, we are at the cusp of rolling out this ambitious project. During the intervening years, a team of almost 100 scientists from most European countries has advanced the GUIDE infrastructure, including scientific tools and methodologies, management and governance structures, technological infrastructures, and operational processes. It is truly exciting to see all of this come together.

The GUIDE Book represents an important part of this journey. It details the research design and makes a strong case for the systematic collection of both objective and subjective data from children, and their parents, over their first 24 years. The GUIDE Book comes at a time when many questions are posed about the future of European economic competitivity, demographic structure, educational performance and health. GUIDE's data will be positioned at the center of these types of policy discussions. The first full waves of GUIDE data collected across Europe will be groundbreaking in themselves. Just imagine how this richness will be enhanced over time from Europe's first cross-national, life-course observatory focusing on children.

December 2025

Gary Pollock
Manchester Metropolitan University
Manchester, UK

Acknowledgments GUIDE has developed through a series of projects funded by the European Commission: MYWeB (GA 613368), the European Cohort Development Project (GA 777449), COORDINATE (GA 101008589), and the current project GUIDEPREP - Growing Up in Digital Europe Preparatory Phase has received funding from the European Union's Horizon Call: HORIZON-INFRA-2021-DEV-02 (Developing and consolidating the European research infrastructures landscape, maintaining global leadership 2021) programme under GA 101078945.

The editors would like to extend a special thanks to Shuang Su for her dedicated work as Editorial Assistant, including administrative coordination, line editing, manuscript preparation, and the creation of the subject index. We are also grateful to Lina Leven for her assistance with formatting, cross-referencing, and standardizing American English spelling.

Competing Interests The editors and authors declare that they have no competing interests.

Contents

Editors and Contributors

About the Editors

Laura K. Taylor (Ph.D.) is a professor in the School of Psychology at University College Dublin. Her research explores the effects of conflict on children's and adolescents' behaviors, including aggression, prosocial actions, and social identity. With more than 20 years of experience in academia and the public sector, she has published more than 110 peer-reviewed works.

Jessica Surdey (Ph.D., M.B.A.) is a research fellow and lecturer at University College Dublin and the Deputy Director of the UCD Centre for the Advancement of Wellbeing in Education. Her research focuses on wellbeing in higher education. She has 16 years of international and interdisciplinary experience in policy, educational practice, and intervention research.

Seaneen Sloan (Ph.D.) is an associate professor in Education at University College Dublin, Deputy Head of the School of Education, Director of the UCD Centre for the Advancement of Wellbeing, and GUIDE Co-Director. She has over 20 years' experience in academic research and has led and supported over 25 research projects on child and youth wellbeing, including longitudinal cohort studies, randomized controlled trials, qualitative and mixed methods studies, and systematic reviews.

Contributors

Toni Babarović Ivo Pilar Institute of Social Sciences, Zagreb, Croatia

Mirta Blažev Ivo Pilar Institute of Social Sciences, Zagreb, Croatia

Arttu Brax Department of Education, University of Helsinki, Helsinki, Finland

Stephanie Cahill Manchester Institute of Education, University of Manchester, Manchester, England;
Policy, Evaluation and Research Unit, Manchester Metropolitan University, Manchester, UK

Iva Černja Rajter Ivo Pilar Institute of Social Sciences, Zagreb, Croatia

Candace Currie University College London, London, UK

Ivan Dević Institute of Social Sciences Ivo Pilar, Zagreb, Croatia

Sabine Düval German Youth Institute, Munich, Germany;
Federal Institute for Population Research, Wiesbaden, Germany

Giulio Ecchia Department of Economics, University of Bologna, Bologna, Italy

Enrico Elefante Italian Youth Agency, Rome, Italy

Eta Krpanec Ivo Pilar Institute of Social Sciences, Zagreb, Croatia

Susanne Kuger German Youth Institute, Munich, Germany;
LMU Munich, Munich, Germany

Gaspar Massiot Institut National d'Etudes Démographiques (INED), Aubervilliers, France

Juliet McEachran Glasgow Caledonian University, London, UK

Gary Pollock Manchester Metropolitan University, Manchester, UK

Giovanni Righetto Department of Economics, University of Bologna, Bologna, Italy

Lynda M. Sagrestano German Youth Institute, Munich, Germany

Hannah Schwarz Department of Political and Social Sciences, Universitat Pompeu Fabra, Barcelona, Spain

Shuang Su School of Education, University College Dublin, Dublin, Ireland

Katja Upadyaya Department of Education, University of Helsinki, Helsinki, Finland

Diana Zavala-Rojas Department of Political and Social Sciences, Universitat Pompeu Fabra, Barcelona, Spain;
European Social Survey ERIC, City St George's, University of London, London, United Kingdom

List of Abbreviations

ALLEA	European Federation of Academies of Sciences and Humanities
ALSPAC	Avon Longitudinal Study of Parents and Children
AOD	Alcohol and Other Drugs
BCS70	British Cohort Study
BiB	Born in Bradford
BMI	Body Mass Index
BMBF	Federal Ministry of Education and Research
BP	Blood Pressure
CAPI	Computer-Assisted Personal Interviewing
CATI	Computer-Assisted Telephone Interviewing
CAVI	Computer-Assisted Video Interviewing
CAWI	Computer-Assisted Web Interviewing
CESSDA	Consortium of European Social Science Data Archives
CFA	Confirmatory Factor Analyses
CFI	Comparative Fit Index
CHRIS	Cooperative Health Research in South Tyrol
COORDINATE	Cohort Community Research and Development Infrastructure Network for Access Throughout Europe
COVID-19	Coronavirus Disease 2019
CRONOS	CROss-National Online Survey (A web-based panel survey run by the ESS)
CRP	C-reactive protein
CST	Core Scientific Team
CTT	Classical Test Theory
DBS	Dried Blood Spots
DDI	Data Documentation Initiative
DEFRA	The UK Department for Environment, Farming and Rural Affairs
DG EMPL	Directorate-General for Employment, Social Affairs and Inclusion

DG RTD	Directorate-General for Research and Innovation
DMHDS	Dunedin Multidisciplinary Health and Development Study
DNA	Deoxyribonucleic acid
DNBC	Danish National Birth Cohort
DOIs	Digital Object Identifiers
DPO	Data Protection Officer
ECLS/ ECLS-K	Early Childhood Longitudinal Studies Program
E. C. D.-G. f. R. a.	European Commission Directorate-General for Research and Innovation
EEA	European Economic Area
EEA	European Education Area
EFA	Exploratory Factor Analyses
ELFE	French Longitudinal Study of Children
EMBS	Ethnic Minority Boost Sample
EOSC	European Open Science Cloud
ERIC	Ethical Research Involving Children
ESRC	Economic and Social Research Council
ESS	European Social Survey
ESS CST	European Social Survey Core Scientific Team
ESS ERIC	European Social Survey European Research Infrastructure Consortium
EU	European Union
EUCOV	European COVID-19
EU-SILC	The European Union Statistics on Income and Living Conditions
FAIR	Findable-Accessible-Interoperable-Reusable
FDZ-LIfBi	Research Data Center at the Leibniz Institute for Educational Trajectories
FIML	Full Information Maximum Likelihood
GATEKEEPER	Smart Living Homes – Whole Interventions Demonstrator for People at Health and Social Risks
GBP	Great Britain Pound
GDP	Gross Domestic Product
GDPR	General Data Protection Regulation
GEMS	Global Enteric Multicenter Study
GenR	Generation R Study
GESIS	Leibniz Institute for the Social Sciences
GGS	The Generation and Gender Survey
GGP	The Generation and Gender Programme
GO FAIR	Global Open FAIR
GUI	Growing Up in Ireland
GUIDE	Growing Up in Digital Europe
GUIDEPREP	Growing Up in Digital Europe Preparation Phase
GWAS	Genome-Wide Association Studies
HBSC	Health Behaviour in School-Aged Children

HCAP	Harmonized Cognitive Assessment Protocol
HELIX	Human Early-Life Exposome study
HPA	Hypothalamus Pituitary Adrenal
IEA	International Association for the Evaluation of Educational Achievement
IEMBS	Immigrant and Ethnic Minority Boost
IL-6	Interleukin 6
IL-2	Interleukin 2
IL-1β	Interleukin 1 beta
Infra4NextGen	Infrastructure for Next Generation (Full project title: Providing research infrastructure services to support Next Generation EU)
IRT	Item Response Theory
ISCED	International Standard Classification of Education
ISO	International Organization for Standardization
ISTAT	Italian National Institute of Statistics
ITC	International Test Commission
JECS	Japan Environment and Children's Study
KABC	Kaufman Assessment Battery for Children
KiGGS	German Health Interview and Examination Survey for Children and Adolescents
LGBTQ+	Lesbian, Gay, Bisexual, Transgender, Queer (or Questioning), and others
LIfBi	Leibniz Institute for Educational Trajectories
LQA	Linguistic Quality Assurance
LSAC	Longitudinal Study of Australian Children
MAR	Missing at Random
MCS	Millennium Cohort Study
MG-CFA	Multi-group Confirmatory Factor Analysis
MoBa	Norwegian Mother, Father and Child Cohort Study
MPISOC	Max Planck Institute for Social Law and Social Policy
MYWeB	Measuring Youth Well-being Project
NEPS	National Educational Panel Study
NGO	Non-Governmental Organization
NHS	National Health Service
NNAT	Naglieri Nonverbal Ability Test
OECD	Organisation for Economic Co-operation and Development
OSF	Open Science Framework
PAUL	Pilot Application in Urban Landscapes (A specific environmental project the ESS contributes to)
PISA	Programme for International Student Assessment
RMSEA	Root Mean Square Error of Approximation
RNA	Ribonucleic acid
RSDs	Responsive Survey Designs
SBI	SHARE Berlin Institute

SDGs	United Nations Sustainable Development Goals
SEED	Study of Early Education and Development
SHARE	Survey of Health, Ageing and Retirement in Europe
SHARE-ERIC	Survey of Health, Ageing and Retirement in Europe – European Research Infrastructure Consortium
SI	Structure of Intellect
SMS	Short Message Service
SRMR	Standardized Root Mean-square Residual
SRS	Simple Random Sampling
SSHOC	Social Sciences and Humanities Open Cloud
SUSTAIN-2	Next Steps in Securing the Sustainability of the European Social Survey (A major EU Horizon 2020 grant project)
SystRS	Systematic Random Sampling
TIMSS	Trends in International Mathematics and Science Study
TL	Telomere Length
TLI	Tucker–Lewis Index
TNF-α	Tumor Necrosis Factor alpha
TRAPD	Translation, Review, Adjudication, Pretesting, and Documentation
UKHLS	Understanding Society: United Kingdom Household Longitudinal Study
UKRI	UK Research and Innovation
UNICEF	United Nations Children's Fund
UNCRC	United Nations Convention on the Rights of the Child
US NIA	United States National Institute on Aging
VMI	Video Mediated Interviews
VO2	Volume of Oxygen
WHO	World Health Organization
WISC	Wechsler Intelligence Scale for Children
YAB	Youth Advisory Board

List of Tables

List of Boxes

Chapter 1
GUIDE's Conceptual Framework for Child Wellbeing in a Digital Age

Jessica Surdey, Seaneen Sloan, and Laura K. Taylor

GUIDE's Approach to Wellbeing

GUIDE aims to track children's wellbeing and psychosocial development across Europe, alongside key indicators from their homes, neighborhoods, and schools. Wellbeing is a complex, multi-dimensional concept understood through quality of life, living conditions, and subjective experiences. Because wellbeing is dynamic and changes over time, measuring it across different developmental periods is inherently complex. Promoting wellbeing is not only vital in childhood but also serves as a foundation for positive outcomes in adulthood. For example, wellbeing has implications across the life course including improved health, relationships, self-esteem, and academic and job performance (Adler et al., 2017; Bogg & Roberts, 2004; Hoyt et al., 2012; Proctor et al., 2010; Ramaj & Pollock, 2025a; Rees et al., 2009; Rowe et al., 2007; Seligman et al., 2009). In short, lower levels of wellbeing in childhood are correlated with individual, social, and societal costs (Layard, 2013).

Wellbeing is integral to health, which is defined by the World Health Organization (WHO) as "a state of complete physical, mental and social wellbeing and not merely the absence of disease or infirmity" (WHO, 1948). Yet, children and adolescents worldwide face increasing vulnerabilities, including poverty, unequal access to education and healthcare, climate change, decreased mental health, violence, and exposure to harmful digital technologies. Economically, over 20% of children lived in relative income poverty in forty of the world's richest countries from 2019 to 2021 (UNICEF, 2023). Worldwide about 23.2% of children under five suffer from stunted height for their age, and in the least developed countries this increases to about 33.9% (WHO, 2025). Beyond physical health, mental wellbeing is a critical concern. One

J. Surdey (✉) · S. Sloan
School of Education, University College Dublin, Dublin, Ireland
e-mail: jessica.surdey@ucd.ie

L. K. Taylor
School of Psychology, University College Dublin, Dublin, Ireland

L. K. Taylor et al. (eds.), *Growing Up in Digital Europe*, Springer Series on Child and Family Studies, https://doi.org/10.1007/978-3-032-30592-3_1

in seven young people between 10 and 19 years of age has a mental disorder (WHO, 2024), suicide is the fourth most significant cause of death for adolescents globally (UNICEF, 2023), and the economic cost of neglecting youth mental health is estimated at around $387.2 billion annually for ages 0 to 19 (UNICEF, 2023). These individual vulnerabilities get more complex with broader systemic crises. Annually, thirty-eight million children experience disruptions to schooling caused by climate change (Save the Children, 2025). Worldwide, 420 million children are living in areas affected by conflict (Graham et al., 2019), and every 5 min a child is killed by violence (UNICEF, 2019). Over half of all children experience physical, sexual, and/or emotional violence every year (Hillis et al., 2016). 2023 marked the highest number of conflicts seen since World War II, driving a record 117 million people from their homes (UNHCR, 2023). Finally, the modern landscape presents new risks: over the past decade, the time children aged 9–16 spend online has nearly doubled, rising from an average of 1.5 h per day to almost 3 h daily (Smahel et al., 2020). Consequently, problematic digital use is increasingly linked with social isolation, sleep deprivation, and attention fragmentation (Haidt, 2024). Despite the growing concerns and issues around these threats to childhood wellbeing, UNICEF reports there are still data gaps (Gromada et al., 2020). To identify and address these issues, GUIDE will map the processes by which these various factors influence childhood wellbeing and development.

GUIDE's Lessons Learned

GUIDE has developed through a series of projects funded by the European Commission: MYWeB, the European Cohort Development Project, COORDINATE, and GUIDEPREP. A Delphi survey conducted as part of the MYWeB project identified two major gaps in wellbeing research: first, a lack of comparable longitudinal data needed to track child development and wellbeing across Europe (Goswami et al., 2016; Pollock et al., 2018); and second, the need to improve the use of standardized measures of subjective wellbeing.

GUIDE's Good Practices

To address these gaps, GUIDE goes beyond traditional economic indicators and considers both material and non-material factors that influence children's overall wellbeing. GUIDE's focus on subjective wellbeing aligns with global priorities, as highlighted by UNICEF's "State of the World's Children" report (UNICEF, 2023). Additionally, GUIDE's longitudinal design will enable measurement that can capture the dynamic and holistic view of children's wellbeing to complement the existing cross-sectional surveys, such as the International Survey of Children's Wellbeing

(Children's Worlds, 2019). With this foundation, GUIDE aims to provide stakeholders and policymakers with a holistic understanding of the conditions and opportunities that affect children's lives throughout development. The data will contribute to policies and interventions that target risk and protective factors to support children to realize their full potential (see Chap. 9 in this book).

GUIDE's data will address critical gaps, providing insights into factors from family, school, and community contexts that influence life satisfaction. GUIDE follows the OECD's framework for *Measuring What Matters for Child Wellbeing and Policies* (OECD, 2021a). More specifically, GUIDE advances a measurement of child wellbeing that:

- is multi-dimensional, encompassing a range of aspects of children's lives,
- reflects children's present and future,
- is age and developmentally situated,
- integrates children's views and perspectives,
- captures children's environments and settings where they grow up, and
- includes related public policies.

Based on its efforts, GUIDE was recognized by the World Happiness Report for its potential to enhance understanding of child and adolescent wellbeing (Helliwell et al., 2024).

GUIDE Is Multi-Disciplinary & Multi-Dimensional

"*Multi-disciplinarity* is at the heart of GUIDE, both in the topics it addresses as well as in the development of alliances across a wide range of professionals" (Ramaj & Pollock, 2025b, p. 4). This approach is reflected in GUIDE's development team, which includes research scientists from sociology, health, psychology, education, public policy, economics, demographic science, family studies, and data sciences.

Children's wellbeing is measured in GUIDE through a *multi-dimensional* approach aligned with the four thematic areas most frequently used in child wellbeing research: material outcomes; physical health outcomes; social, emotional, and cultural outcomes; and cognitive development and educational outcomes (Fernandes et al., 2012; OECD, 2021a). These thematic areas are examined across four major domains of children's lives: home and family life; school or early care life; social and community life; and online or digital life. To assess these areas and domains, GUIDE uses multiple indicators, including a combination of self-reported measures of wellbeing with other (objective and subjective) domain-specific measures (see Chap. 5 in this book; Children's Worlds, 2019; Goswami et al., 2016; Pollock et al., 2021; Stiglitz et al., 2009). In sum, GUIDE's multi-dimensional approach provides rich and detailed insight into the ways people live their lives, helping to form a holistic picture of child wellbeing and development (Bradshaw & Richardson, 2009; Fernandes et al., 2012; OECD, 2015, 2021a).

GUIDE's Wellbeing Model

GUIDE's wellbeing model (Fig. 1.1) is rooted in Bronfenbrenner's ecological systems theory of lifespan development, which emphasizes the interrelationship of different developmental processes (e.g., cognitive, social, biological) with the environment and cultural context (Bronfenbrenner, 1979; Bronfenbrenner & Ceci, 1994; Bronfenbrenner et al., 1986; Garbarino, 2014). Although GUIDE's wellbeing model involves both objective and subjective measures of wellbeing, it places a special focus on *subjective wellbeing*, that is, the individual child's perspective on their personality, abilities, aims, expectations, social comparisons, online lives, needs, and relationships. These factors are examined alongside other economic, social, and psychological factors.

In the GUIDE wellbeing model, the individual (child) is viewed as the center of the system and as an active contributor to their family, community, and society. At the *individual* level, there are diverse developmental factors contributing to wellbeing, such as the child's biology, cognitive development, identity, and emotions. The *microsystem* includes the daily activities and relationships closest to the child, most often associated with family and peers. The *mesosystem* is the resources and networks surrounding the child in their communities, such as the larger school environment. The *macrosystem* is the context and policies that shape the child's environment; these factors are often filtered through the other more proximal levels to the individual child. Each of these levels are part of the *chronosystem*, which recognizes lifespan development as a time-dependent process with cumulative effects over time. The complexity of understanding child wellbeing necessitates studying

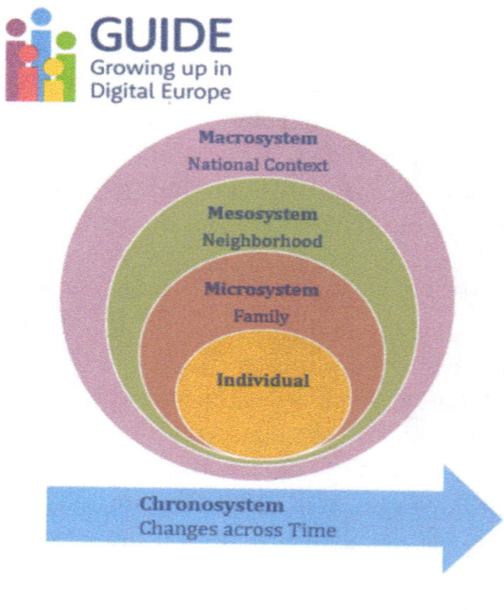

Fig. 1.1 GUIDE's wellbeing model, adapted from Bronfenbrenner (1979)

multiple outcomes, stakeholders, domains, and systems, which themselves are interdependent, connected, and linked in a multi-directional, interactive web of drivers and determinants.

Drawing on Bronfenbrenner's framework, wellbeing emerges from dynamic, reciprocal interactions between children and their environments, across multiple layers of context. This perspective is enriched by insights from sociology, education, health, and social policy research. These perspectives collectively highlight how social structures and institutions mediate opportunities and inequalities across the life course. By combining these perspectives, GUIDE captures both the proximal influences of everyday life and the wider forces of social change that shape children's trajectories.

Individual

GUIDE focuses on the child's biological (see Chap. 7 in this book), psychological, and developmental capacities. Questionnaires thus capture domains such as physical health, nutrition, sleep, activity, and healthcare use, alongside psychological and emotional wellbeing, including happiness, life satisfaction, loneliness, and coping. This primary data is further enriched by information from caregivers on pregnancy and birth, early child development, and health behaviors. Consistent with Bronfenbrenner's emphasis on the child as an active agent, GUIDE recognizes that children not only experience but also shape their environments through their temperament, coping styles, and decision-making processes that influence relationships and outcomes.

Microsystem

The microsystem encompasses the context of daily life where children's immediate interactions occur (e.g., family, peers, school, digital contexts). GUIDE collects data on parent–child relationships, parenting styles, conflict and support, and family activities. Children's experiences with friends and peers are also captured, including trust, belonging, and bullying, while school is addressed as both a site of learning and a social environment. These domains reflect how the quality of close interactions lays the foundation for wellbeing, and how differences in these experiences can set children on divergent developmental paths.

Mesosystem

The mesosystem refers to the linkages between microsystems, including networks and settings surrounding the child in their communities. In GUIDE, this is operationalized through measures of parental employment and working conditions, socioeconomic resources, housing, neighborhood cohesion, and community safety. For instance, a parent's job security or stress may affect the quality of family interactions, while the availability of healthcare or safe play spaces in the community shapes children's opportunities. These indirect influences are critical in understanding the ecology of wellbeing, as they demonstrate how the wider environment can support or undermine family functioning and, in turn, children's outcomes. By capturing these cross-setting interactions, GUIDE acknowledges that wellbeing depends not only on the quality of individual environments, but also on the strength and alignment of the bridges between them.

Macrosystem

At the macrosystem level, GUIDE examines the broader cultural, political, and institutional systems that shape childhood. This includes the welfare regimes, education systems, and policy structures of participating countries, as well as cultural values and social attitudes. Questionnaire modules on values, political socialization, and children's rights and voice allow GUIDE to capture how these macro-level factors filter into children's everyday lives (see Chap. 5 in this book). By harmonizing data across countries, GUIDE enables comparative analysis of how different welfare and policy contexts influence wellbeing, inequalities, and opportunities for children across Europe (see Chap. 9 in this book).

Chronosystem

Finally, all these levels are embedded within the chronosystem, which situates development in time. GUIDE's longitudinal design, following children up to age 24, allows researchers to trace how wellbeing changes across key transitions, such as adolescence, school transitions, and entry into adulthood. By collecting repeated measures across waves, GUIDE is uniquely positioned to trace how children's health, relationships, education, and opportunities evolve over the life course, and how early experiences accumulate to shape later outcomes.

GUIDE's wellbeing model serves as the foundation for a broad range of research questions, underpinned by a multi-national, comparative longitudinal approach (see Table 1.1).

Table 1.1 Mapping research questions onto guide's wellbeing model

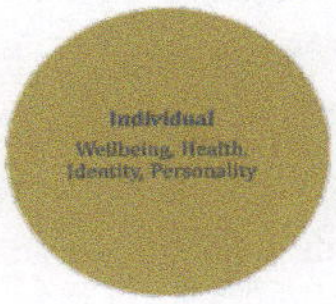	Cognitive development, material goods and services, physical health and development, and wellbeing **Research Questions:** How does social engagement impact child wellbeing? What social, emotional, and psychological challenges do children face, and how do these challenges affect their overall wellbeing? How can a child's ________ impact their wellbeing across Europe? (e.g., nationality, ethnicity, citizenship, gender, disability, social class, sexuality, etc.) How does dental behavior for children influence their health outcomes? How does physical health in childhood impact wellbeing into adolescence?
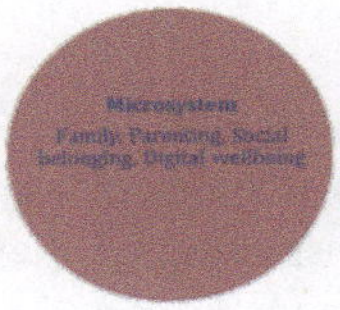	Relationships and activities including family life, friends, leisure, play, and usage of digital devices **Research Questions:** How do parental practices and their impact on child wellbeing differ across European contexts? How do parental wellbeing and lifestyle influence the development and wellbeing of children? How does differential access to digital devices affect child wellbeing? How do family structures differ across Europe, how are different family structures associated with child wellbeing outcomes? Do changes to family structure impact their later wellbeing?
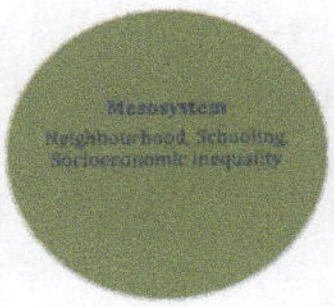	Resources and networks including school and neighborhood **Research Questions:** How do differences in neighborhoods across Europe impact child wellbeing? How do different educational experiences across Europe influence educational outcomes? What are the key drivers? How do drivers of social inequality differ across Europe, how do they impact child wellbeing? How does parental employment status across Europe impact child wellbeing and educational outcomes?
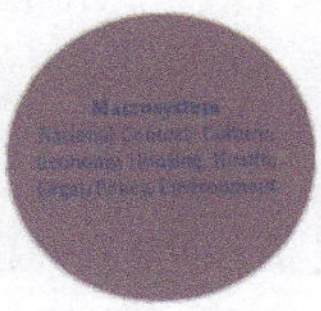	Context and child-relevant policy, such as family, housing, health, education, and care **Research Questions:** How do country characteristics, such as access to public schools, free medical care, etc., affect child development across Europe? How does access to health care across Europe influence children's physical health? How do different levels of digital access to information affect children's later civic engagement?

(continued)

Table 1.1 (continued)

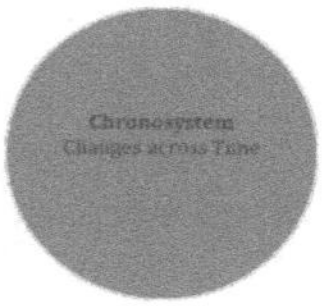	Lifespan development is a time-dependent process with cumulative effects over time **Research Questions:** How does child wellbeing at an early age impact the trajectory of their future wellbeing? What measures can be used as predictors of child wellbeing from an early age to adulthood? Are there cohort effects, comparing children in the birth and 8-year-old cohorts? Are there generational differences, comparing children and parents?

GUIDE's Core Elements

GUIDE's wellbeing model and research questions are advanced through three key aspects: a child-centered approach rooted in youth's voices, cross-national and longitudinal comparative power, and exploring the digital landscape in childhood.

Child Centered and Youth Voice

First, young people, their voices and perspectives, are at the heart of GUIDE (Goswami et al., 2016; Pollock et al., 2018). Including children as active agents whose perspectives can be heard in matters concerning them in policy, practice and research is gaining momentum.

Reflecting this best practice, youth advisory boards (YABs) were essential actors informing the development of GUIDE instruments and fieldwork processes (Ramaj & Pollock, 2025a). For example, YABs established in Finland, Croatia, England, and Portugal played a key role in reviewing the GUIDE study procedures and questionnaire development (see Chap. 5 in this book). Advisors, aged 14 to 34, were selected from diverse backgrounds to represent various ethnicities, religions, and socioeconomic groups, with efforts to balance age and gender, and participated in a series of workshops. The first workshop introduced the GUIDE study and allowed youth advisors to suggest improvements regarding interview duration, location, rapport-building strategies, caregiver involvement, and participant incentives. The second workshop focused on reviewing the questionnaire, where advisors identified complex or redundant questions and suggested ways to make it more accessible for younger respondents. In the final workshop, advisors evaluated the feasibility of interviewing children as young as eight, recommending child-friendly adaptations, casual introductions, and comfortable interview settings. Advisors' insights were instrumental in making the GUIDE questionnaire more inclusive, accessible, and responsive to young participants' needs. Such engagement will continue to ensure that children's perspectives are taken into account, reflecting GUIDE's recognition that young people are experts in their own lives and should be involved in research that concerns them.

Cross-National, Longitudinal Comparative Power

Second, GUIDE has two strategic advantages over existing approaches to child wellbeing: it is both cross-national and longitudinal. At the cross-national level, international instruments such as the OECD Program for International Student Assessment (PISA) and the WHO Health Behavior in School-Aged Children (HBSC) survey have helped advance what we know and understand about child wellbeing at different points in a range of areas. For example, in the HBSC, which assesses adolescent health and wellbeing every four years, young people are asked to rate their life satisfaction using a visual ladder scale, indicating the ladder step at which they would place their lives at present (Cosma et al., 2023). The HSBC has comparative power across 44 countries, but this single item does not fully capture the nuance of subjective wellbeing. Similarly, PISA assesses wellbeing using questions surrounding life satisfaction for 15-year-olds. In particular, PISA asks "How satisfied are you with each of the following?" with respect to ten domains: (1) What you learn at school, (2) Your relationship with your teachers, (3) Your life at school, (4) The way that you look, (5) How you use your time, (6) Your health, (7) Your relationship with your parents/guardians, (8) The neighborhood you live in, (9) The friends you have, and (10) All the things you have (OECD, 2023). Although this approach captures subjective wellbeing in multiple domains across 81 countries, deeper understandings are limited because it considers only a single time point and only one age; the *development* of wellbeing cannot be examined, which can be teased out across longitudinal and cohort designs.

At the same time, individual countries have embarked on efforts to capture longitudinal data on child wellbeing. For example, during the COVID-19 pandemic, cohort surveys such as Born in Bradford (BiB), Danish National Birth Cohort (DNBC), and Growing Up in Ireland (GUI) revealed the national effects of lockdowns on children, young people, and families. BiB highlighted increased maternal depression and anxiety, especially among isolated and financially insecure mothers (McEachan et al., 2024). DNBC identified vulnerable adolescents, particularly those in crowded homes or without outdoor space, showing temporary declines in mental health (Strandberg-Larsen et al., 2025). GUI found high depressive symptoms among Irish youth, with notable gender differences. These findings helped shape public health responses and mental health strategies, underline the value of longitudinal data in addressing complex, evolving social challenges, and inform holistic, scientifically grounded policy design (Kelly et al., 2023). However, cross-national comparison is limited because of the lack of harmonization, including distinct measurement, data collection modes, ages, and waves.

Existing child cohort studies illustrate the powerful potential for a pan-European cohort study on child wellbeing. Such harmonized cross-national designs enable new scientific advances. This coordinated approach is critical because research has persistently shown that early life experiences have a clear effect on later life outcomes, and GUIDE's longitudinal and cross-national design means it will be able to give valuable information to understand and promote child wellbeing and positive life trajectories.

GUIDE's comparative longitudinal data will allow hypotheses to be tested by accounting for multi-level contexts, particularly national ones, as well as tracing experiences over time. This unique data would facilitate increasingly internationalized policies on education, health, and family, particularly in the earliest years of life. Crucially, there is no comparable longitudinal data source currently available to inform such policies. As the GUIDE respondents develop, an increasing body of data will indicate the precise impact of national policies and pinpoint where interventions are needed. In sum, GUIDE will be directly relevant to European and international policy initiatives and frameworks, such as the European Child Guarantee, the European Pillar of Social Rights, the Sustainable Development Goals, and the UN Convention on the Rights of the Child.

Exploring the Digital Landscape in Childhood

Third, childhood today is shaped by the digital revolution. GUIDE tackles digital challenges, and opportunities, head on. Over the past decade, the time children aged 9–16 spend online has nearly doubled, rising from an average of 1.5 h per day to almost 3 h daily (Smahel et al., 2020). Regular access and more screen time increases the likelihood of encountering harmful content, and it can also negatively affect attention span (Haidt, 2024). More time spent online for children also means they engage less in physical activity and real-world social interactions, which could lead to worse physical and mental health outcomes (Burns & Gottschalk, 2019; OECD, 2018, 2021b). Greater time spent on social media has been linked to negative body image, distress, depression, and suicidal ideation (Kelly et al., 2018; Twenge et al., 2025; Vidal et al., 2020). Problematic digital use may lead to significant negative outcomes across multiple domains, such as social deprivation, disordered sleep, attention fragmentation, and addiction (Haidt, 2024).

At the same time, technology is an integral part of children's lives, impacting various aspects of their wellbeing; it can improve lives, facilitating communication, education, and leisure (Van Deursen & Helsper, 2018). Children today are digital natives, and rather than adopting a risk-focused perspective, a proactive approach is necessary to promote young people's digital skill development and ensure safe participation, because digital technology is not going away (Livingstone, 2024; Vissenberg et al., 2022). Digital environments can support positive youth development through overcoming barriers and challenges to traditional help-seeking with mental health and online counselling; they can also support enhanced accessibility and cost-effectiveness, and reduce the stigmatizing effects of poor mental health (Tibbs et al., 2022). In short, GUIDE adopts a balanced, nuanced approach to exploring the digital landscape in childhood, investigating both its positive and negative effects on wellbeing across Europe.

Box 1.1. Digital Life: Key Case Ireland

To demonstrate the utility of GUIDE's approach, we focus on social interaction and online safety among children in Ireland (Mohan, 2023a). Online safety has been a key agenda for policymakers, particularly concerning bullying, gambling, abuse, exposure to harmful content, and problematic use among internet users. The 2021 National Survey on Online Safety with children (9–17 years), parents, and adults in Ireland highlights the critical need for continued efforts to enhance online safety. The report reveals widespread exposure and risk: 62% of children use social media. 13% of children and one in five (21%) of 15–17-year-olds have experienced something that made them feel uncomfortable or scared. Furthermore, over one-third of 20-year-olds surveyed in 2018–2019 met an online virtual contact in person. Adolescents aged 13–14 experienced online and offline bullying more than other age groups. Gender also plays a role in the results; for example, girls engage more with their parents on online safety. Evidence also suggests conflict between parents appears to be a risk factor for excessive internet use (Mohan, 2023b) and two-thirds of 17–18-year-olds reported at least one symptom of excessive internet use with impact on their wellbeing (O'Reilly & Mohan, 2023). Simultaneously, online gambling has become more prevalent in Ireland, and the link between childhood experiences of gambling and problem gambling in adulthood (Ó Ceallaigh et al., 2024) has been identified. These findings underscore a critical gap: the National Advisory Council for Online Safety (2021) survey revealed no long-term data tracking or online safety protections for children and young people in Ireland.

Evidence for Future Policy

GUIDE data will capture time spent online during schooldays and weekends, types of devices available at home, access to these devices, frequency of engagement in specific online activities, parental monitoring levels, permitted activities, challenges encountered with online tools, and emotional responses related to device usage across different age groups. This comprehensive dataset will support informed policy decisions aimed at enhancing online safety measures and addressing evolving trends in digital behavior.

GUIDE data will also enable researchers to identify factors that mediate the negative outcomes of digital engagement. Variables such as parental communication, emotional factors, social norms, socio-economic status, and the educational environment will be examined as risk factors. Monitoring the direct and indirect factors longitudinally would also enable the observation of contextual changes, facilitating the adjustment of policy implications over time, especially in comparison to other European countries. Open-access, cross-culturally comparative, and continuous monitoring of children will support the design of evidence-based policies and interventions for the challenges children and caregivers experience online.

Given the children's digital landscape, GUIDE will yield policy insights not only for Ireland, which recently became one of the 70 members of WePROTECT Global Alliance in 2016 to prevent online child sexual abuse, but also across Europe. For example, GUIDE data could be used to monitor and compare the implementation of the EU Digital Strategy, including the Digital Services Act and the proposed Digital Fairness Act. Such data files are crucial to fill the void of comparative, longitudinal data on children's digital engagement and wellbeing in this evolving policy context.

GUIDE Book: Cross-National Longitudinal Research on Child Wellbeing

In this book we document the scientific methodology of GUIDE. Throughout the chapters, key cases are presented to illustrate best practices by using national examples (e.g., Ireland, Germany, France, Norway, and Slovenia) of cross-cutting or common cases with variation in terms of national characteristics (e.g., size, GDP), participation in European cross-national surveys (e.g., ESS, PISA), and practical considerations related to the history of GUIDE. We hope this volume provides a roadmap for the first wave of GUIDE and other cross-national, longitudinal studies for the scientific community.

- This Chapter (Surdey et al., 2026): GUIDE's Conceptual Framework for Studying Child Wellbeing in a Digital Age focuses on GUIDE's overarching multidisciplinary conceptual perspective, research questions, child-centered approach, and consideration of the digital transformation of the last 25 years.
- Chapter 2 (Cahill, 2026): Ethical Considerations for Cross-National, Longitudinal Research with Children and Families covers ethics for GUIDE given the focus on children's wellbeing on issues such as GDPR, data privacy, informed consent, protection of participants, and international best practices from cohort studies.
- Chapter 3 (Upadyaya et al., 2026): Managing Fieldwork Across Contexts covers practical aspects of data collection, modes, and methods for studying child wellbeing.
- Chapter 4 (Massiot & Su, 2026): Selecting and Retaining Representative Longitudinal Infant and Child Cohort Samples covers the GUIDE panel design, learned from best practices in sampling and recruitment strategies, weighting and consideration of diverse, hard-to-reach samples.
- Chapter 5 (Babarović et al., 2026): Developing a Cross-National, Longitudinal Questionnaire to Study Child Wellbeing explores how the GUIDE survey instruments were developed, validated, and adapted for diverse populations.
- Chapter 6 (Černja Rajter et al., 2026): Cognitive Assessment in Children covers the development of GUIDE's bespoke cognitive data measure.
- Chapter 7 (McEachran & Currie, 2026): Possibilities and Considerations for Biological Data Collection with Children Across Contexts explores methods for collecting and storing biological data and the ethical, financial, technical, and feasibility challenges related to the study's research aims.
- Chapter 8 (Zavala-Rojas & Schwarz, 2026): Open Science in Longitudinal Cohort Designs with Children introduces key principles of FAIR and GDPR as frameworks guiding GUIDE's approach to open science.
- Chapter 9 (Düval et al., 2026): Best Practices for Data Harmonization and Comparability of Child Wellbeing across Europe focuses on ensuring that the study is comparable and harmonized across various cultural and national contexts.

- Chapter 10 (Righetto et al., 2026): Making Ends Meet, the Funding of Cross-National Cohort Studies addresses the financial aspects of conducting a large-scale study, covering funding sources, cost management, and financial sustainability over the long term.

Growing Up in Digital Europe: GUIDE's Cross-National Longitudinal Research on Child Wellbeing is a must-have resource for researchers, professors, and graduate students as well as policy makers, educators, and related professionals in child, school, and developmental psychology, social work, public health, epidemiology, demography, human development and family studies, social psychology, sociology, and communication.

References

Adler, A., Unanue, W., Osin, E., Ricard, M., Alkire, S., & Seligman, M. (2017). Psychological well-being. In Centre for Bhutan Studies and Gross National Happiness (Eds.), *Happiness: Transforming the development landscape* (pp. 118–155). The Centre for Bhutan Studies.

Babarović, T., Krpanec, E., Blažev, M., & Černja Rajter, I. (2026). Chapter 5: Developing a cross-national, longitudinal questionnaire to study child well-being. In L. K. Taylor, J. F. Surdey & S. Sloan (Eds.), *Growing Up in digital Europe: GUIDE's cross-national longitudinal research on child well-being* (pp. 67–84). Springer.

Bogg, T., & Roberts, B. W. (2004). Conscientiousness and health-related behaviours: A meta-analysis of the leading behavioural contributors to mortality. *Psychology Bulletin,130*, 887–919.

Bradshaw, J., & Richardson, D. (2009). An index of child well-being in Europe. *Child Indicators Research,2*(3), 319–351. https://doi.org/10.1007/s12187-009-9037-7

Bronfenbrenner, U. (1979). *The ecology of human development: Experiments by nature and design.* Harvard University Press.

Bronfenbrenner, U., et al. (1986). Ecology of the family as a context for human development: Research perspectives. *Developmental Psychology,22*(6), 723–742. https://doi.org/10.1037/0012-1649.22.6.723

Bronfenbrenner, U., & Ceci, S. (1994). Nature-nurture reconceptualized in developmental perspective: A bioecological model. *Psychological Review,101*(4), 568–586. https://doi.org/10.1037/0033-295X.101.4.568

Burns, T., & Gottschalk, F. (Eds.). (2019). *Educating 21st century children: Emotional well-being in the digital age.* OECD Publishing. https://doi.org/10.1787/b7f33425-en

Cahill, S. (2026). Chapter 2: Ethical considerations for cross-national, longitudinal research with children and families. In L. K. Taylor, J. F. Surdey & S. Sloan (Eds.), *Growing up in digital Europe: GUIDE's cross-national longitudinal research on child well-being* (pp. 19–35). Springer.

Černja Rajter, I., Babarović, T., & Dević, I. (2026). Chapter 6: Cognitive assessment in children. In L. K. Taylor, J. F. Surdey & S. Sloan (Eds.), *Growing up in digital Europe: GUIDE's cross-national longitudinal research on child well-being* (pp. 85–99). Springer.

Children's Worlds. (2019). *International survey of children's well-being.* https://www.isciweb.org

Cosma, A., Abdrakhmanova, S., Taut, D., Schrijvers, K., Catunda, C., & Schnohr, C. (2023). *A focus on adolescent mental health and well-being in Europe, central Asia and Canada: Health behaviour in school-aged children international report from the 2021/2022 survey* (Vol. 1). WHO Regional Office for Europe. https://iris.who.int/bitstreams/2e2d0d63-bd03-4c9d-aec5-64bb161bf98b/download

Düval, S., Kuger, S., & Sagrestano, L. M. (2026). Chapter 9: Best practices for data harmonization and comparability of child wellbeing across Europe. In L. K. Taylor, J. F. Surdey & S. Sloan (Eds.), *Growing up in digital Europe: GUIDE's cross-national longitudinal research on child well-being* (pp. 155–175). Springer.

Fernandes, L., Mendes, A., & Teixeira, A. (2012). A review essay on the measurement of child well-being. *Social Indicators Research*. https://doi.org/10.1007/s11205-011-9814-9

Garbarino, J. (2014). Ecological perspective on child well-being. In A. Ben-Arieh, F. Casas, I. Frønes & J. E. Korbin (Eds.), *Handbook of child well-being: Theories, methods and policies in global perspective*. Springer. https://doi.org/10.1007/978-90-481-9063-8_140

Goswami, H., Fox, C., & Pollock, G. (2016). The current evidence base and future needs in improving children's well-being across Europe: Is there a case for a comparative longitudinal survey? *Child Indicators Research,9*(2), 371–388. https://doi.org/10.1007/s12187-015-9323-5

Graham, G., Kirollos, M., Knag Fylkesnes, G., Salarkia, K., & Wong, N. (2019). *Stop the war on children: Protecting children in 21st century conflict*. https://resourcecentre.savethechildren.net/document/stop-war-children-protecting-children-21st-centuryconflict/

Gromada, A., Rees, G., & Chzhen, Y. (2020). *Worlds of influence: Understanding what shapes child well-being in rich countries*. UNICEF. https://www.unicef.org/reports/worlds-influence-what-shapes-child-well-being-rich-countries-2020

Haidt, J. (2024). *The anxious generation: How the great rewiring of childhood is causing an epidemic of mental illness*. Penguin.

Helliwell, J. F., Huang, H., Shiplett, H., & Wang, S. (2024). Happiness of the younger, the older, and those in between. In J. F. Helliwell, R. Layard, J. D. Sachs, J.-E. De Neve, L. B. Aknin & S. Wang (Eds.), *World happiness report 2024* (Chap. 2). Wellbeing Research Centre, University of Oxford. https://doi.org/10.18724/whr-f1p2-qj33

Hillis, S., Mercy, J., Amobi, A., & Kress, H. (2016). Global prevalence of past-year violence against children: A systematic review and minimum estimates. *Pediatrics, 137*(3). https://doi.org/10.1542/peds.2015-4079

Hoyt, L. T., Chase-Lansdale, P. L., McDade, T. W., & Adam, E. K. (2012). Positive youth, healthy adults: Does positive well-being in adolescence predict better perceived health and fewer risky health behaviours in young adulthood? *Journal of Adolescent Health,50*, 66–73.

Kelly, L., Murray, A., Quail, A., & McNamara, E. (2023). Adaptations to a cohort study in response to the COVID-19 pandemic: Insights from growing up in Ireland. *Longitudinal and Life Course Studies, 14*(2), 294–307. https://bristoluniversitypressdigital.com/view/journals/llcs/14/2/article-p294.xml

Kelly, Y., Zilanawala, A., Booker, C., & Sacker, A. (2018). Social media use and adolescent mental health: Findings from the UK Millennium cohort study. *eClinicalMedicine, 6*, 59–68. https://doi.org/10.1016/J.ECLINM.2018.12.005

Layard, R. (2013). Mental health: The new frontier for labour economics. *IZA Journal of Labor Policy,2*, 1–16. https://doi.org/10.1186/2193-9004-2-2

Livingstone, S. (2024). Reflections on the meaning of "digital" in research on adolescents' digital lives. *Journal of Adolescence,96*(4), 886–891. https://doi.org/10.1002/jad.12322

Massiot, G., & Su, S. (2026). Chapter 4: Selecting and retaining representative longitudinal infant and child cohort samples. In L. K. Taylor, J. F. Surdey & S. Sloan (Eds.), *Growing up in digital Europe: GUIDE's cross-national longitudinal research on child well-being* (pp. 53–66). Springer.

McEachan, R. R. C., Santorelli, G., Watmuff, A., Mason, D., Barber, S. E., Bingham, D. D., Bird, P. K., Lennon, L., Lewer, D., Mon-Williams, M., Shire, K. A., Waiblinger, D., West, J., Yang, T. C., Lawlor, D. A., Pickett, K. E., & Wright, J. (2024). Cohort profile update: Born in Bradford. *International Journal of Epidemiology, 53*(2), Article dyae037. https://doi.org/10.1093/ije/dyae037

McEachran, J., & Currie, C. (2026). Chapter 7: Beyond self-report—Possibilities and considerations for biological data collection with children across contexts. In L. K. Taylor, J. F. Surdey & S.

Sloan (Eds.), *Growing Up in digital Europe: GUIDE's cross-national longitudinal research on child well-being* (pp. 101–135). Springer.

Mohan, G. (2023a). Characteristics and behaviours of young people who meet online contacts face-to-face. *International Journal of Adolescence and Youth, 28*(1), Article 2241524. https://doi.org/10.1080/02673843.2023.2241524

Mohan, G. (2023b). *Factors influencing excessive Internet use among adolescents in Ireland* (ESRI Research Bulletin 2023/08). https://www.esri.ie/publications/factors-influencing-excessive-internet-use-among-adolescents-in-ireland

National Advisory Council for Online Safety. (2021). *Report of a national survey of children, their parents and adults regarding online safety 2021*. https://assets.gov.ie/204409/b9ab5dbd-8fdc-4f97-abfc-a88afb2f6e6f.pdf

OECD. (2015). How's life? 2015: Measuring well-being. *OECD Publishing*. https://doi.org/10.1787/how_life-2015-en

OECD. (2018). *Children and young people's mental health in the digital age*. OECD. http://www.oecd.org/els/health-systems/Children-and-Young-People-Mental-Health-in-the-Digital-Age.pdf

OECD. (2021a). Measuring what matters for child well-being and policies. *OECD Publishing*. https://doi.org/10.1787/e82fded1-en

OECD. (2021b). *Children in the digital environment: Revised typology of risks* (OECD Digital Economy Papers No. 302). OECD Publishing. https://doi.org/10.1787/9b8f222e-en

OECD. (2023). PISA 2022 results (Volume II): Learning during—and from—disruption. *OECD Publishing*. https://doi.org/10.1787/a97db61c-en

Ó Ceallaigh, D., Timmons, S., Robertson, D., & Lunn, P. (2024). *Childhood gambling experiences and adult problem gambling*. https://www.esri.ie/publications/childhood-gambling-experiences-and-adult-problem-gambling

O'Reilly, C., & Mohan, G. (2023). Parental influences on excessive internet use among adolescents. *Internet Research,33*(7), 86–110.

Pollock, G., Goswami, H., & Szymczyk, A. (2021). Child well-being across the life course: What do we know, what should we know? In P. Banati (Ed.), *Sustainable human development across the life course: Evidence from longitudinal research* (pp. 165–192). Bristol University Press. https://doi.org/10.46692/9781529204834.009

Pollock, G., Ozan, J., Goswami, H., & Fox, C. (2018). With a view towards the future: Different options to measure the well-being of children and young people across Europe longitudinally. In G. Pollock, J. Ozan, H. Goswami, G. Rees & A. Stasulane (Eds.), *Measuring youth well-being: How a Pan-European longitudinal survey could improve policy*. Springer.

Proctor, C., Linley, P. A., & Maltby, J. (2010). Very happy youths: Benefits of very high life satisfaction among adolescents. *Social Indicators Research,98*(3), 519–532. https://doi.org/10.1007/s11205-009-9562-2

Ramaj, K., & Pollock, G. (2025a). Growing up in digital Europe (GUIDE): A comparative longitudinal study for child well-being. *European Psychologist,30*(3), 202–212. https://doi.org/10.1027/1016-9040/a000542

Ramaj, K., & Pollock, G. (2025b). Youth Advisory Boards (YABs): The case of growing up in digital Europe (GUIDE). In Z. H. Bíró, E. Çela, P. Krasztev, F. Sipos & E. Xhemi (Eds.), *Equity in education: A handbook for participative approaches in research and development to address school inequalities* (pp. 126–145). CEEOL Press. https://www.ceeol.com/search/chapter-detail?id=1303223

Rees, G., Bradshaw, J., Goswami, H., & Keung, A. (2009). *Understanding children's well-Being: A national survey of young people's well-being*. The Children's Society.

Righetto, G., Ecchia, G., & Elefante, E. (2026). Chapter 10: Making ends meet—Funding and national frameworks of cross-national cohort studies. In L. K. Taylor, J. F. Surdey & S. Sloan (Eds.), *Growing up in digital Europe: GUIDE's cross-national longitudinal research on child well-being* (pp. 177–193). Springer.

Rowe, G., Hirsh, J. B., Anderson, A. K., & Smith, E. E. (2007). Positive affect increases the breadth of attentional selection. *PNAS Proceedings of the National Academy of Sciences of the United States of America,104*, 383–438.

Save the Children. (2025). *Climate change is a grave threat to children's survival*. https://www.savethechildren.org/us/what-we-do/emergency-response/climate-change

Seligman, M. E. P., Ernst, R. M., Gillham, J., Reivich, K., & Linkins, M. (2009). Positive education: Positive psychology and classroom interventions. *Oxford Review of Education,35*(3), 293–311. https://doi.org/10.1080/03054980902934563

Smahel, D., Machackova, H., Mascheroni, G., Dedkova, L., Staksrud, E., Ólafsson, K., Livingstone, S., & Hasebrink, U. (2020). *EU kids online 2020: Survey results from 19 countries*. EU Kids Online. https://doi.org/10.21953/lse.47fdeqj01ofo

Stiglitz, J. E., Sen, A., & Fitoussi, J.-P. (2009). *Report by the commission on the measurement of economic performance and social progress*. http://citeseerx.ist.psu.edu/viewdoc/download?doi=10.1.1.215.58&rep=rep1&type=pdf

Strandberg-Larsen, K., Cederkvist, L., Aakjær, A., Bjerregaard, A. A., Brix, N., Feenstra, B., Meder, I. K., Nohr, E. A., Olsen, S. F., Tøttenborg, S. S., Høst Ramlau-Hansen, C., Vangsted, A. M., & Andersen, A. M. N. (2025). Cohort profile: The Danish National Birth Cohort from foetal life to young adulthood. *International Journal of Epidemiology, 54*(4), Article dyaf083. https://doi.org/10.1093/ije/dyaf083.

Surdey, J. F., Sloan, S., & Taylor, L. K. (2026). Chapter 1: GUIDE's conceptual framework for studying child wellbeing in a digital age. In L. K. Taylor, J. F. Surdey & S. Sloan (Eds.), *Growing up in digital Europe: GUIDE's cross-national longitudinal research on child well-being* (pp. 1–17). Springer.

Tibbs, M., O'Reilly, A., Dwan O'Reilly, M., & Fitzgerald, A. (2022). Online synchronous chat counselling for young people aged 12–25: A mixed methods systematic review protocol. *BMJ Open, 12*(4), Article e061084. https://doi.org/10.1136/bmjopen-2022-061084

Twenge, J., et al. (2025). Social media and depressive symptoms. In *Handbook of children and screens* (pp. 137–140). https://doi.org/10.1007/978-3-031-69362-5_19

UNHCR. (2023). *Global trends report 2023*. https://www.unhcr.org/global-trends-report-2023

UNICEF. (2019). *29 million babies born into conflict in 2018*. https://www.unicef.org/pressreleases/29-million-babies-born-conflict-2018

UNICEF. (2023). *Child poverty in the midst of wealth* (Innocenti Report Card 18). UNICEF Innocenti global office of research and foresight. https://www.unicef.org/innocenti/reports/child-poverty-midst-wealth

Upadyaya, K., Huttunen, I., & Cahill, S. (2026). Chapter 3: Managing fieldwork across contexts—Modes and methods for studying child wellbeing. In L. K. Taylor, J. F. Surdey & S. Sloan (Eds.), *Growing up in digital Europe: GUIDE's cross-national longitudinal research on child well-being* (pp. 37–52). Springer.

Van Deursen, A. J., & Helsper, E. J. (2018). Collateral benefits of internet use: Explaining the diverse outcomes of engaging with the internet. *New Media & Society,20*(7), 2333–2351. https://doi.org/10.1177/1461444817715282

Vidal, C., et al. (2020). Social media use and depression in adolescents: A scoping review. *International Review of Psychiatry,32*(3), 235. https://doi.org/10.1080/09540261.2020.1720623

Vissenberg, J., d'Haenens, L., & Livingstone, S. (2022). Digital literacy and online resilience as facilitators of young people's well-being? *European Psychologist*. https://doi.org/10.1027/1016-9040/a000478

World Health Organization. (1948). Constitution of the world health organization. Retrieved 2026: https://www.who.int/about/governance/constitution

World Health Organization. (2024). *Global Health Data Exchange (GHDx)*. Institute of health metrics and evaluation. https://ghdx.healthdata.org/global-health-data-exchange

World Health Organization. (2025). *Levels and trends in child malnutrition: Key findings of the 2025 edition of the Joint Child Malnutrition Estimates*. World Health Organization. https://iris.who.int/handle/10665/381846

Zavala-Rojas, D., & Schwarz, H. (2026). Chapter 8: Open science in longitudinal, cohort designs with children. In L. K. Taylor, J. F. Surdey & S. Sloan (Eds.), *Growing up in digital Europe: GUIDE's cross-national longitudinal research on child well-being* (pp. 137–153). Springer.

Jessica Surdey (Ph.D., M.B.A.) is a research fellow and lecturer at University College Dublin and the Deputy Director of the UCD Centre for the Advancement of Wellbeing in Education. Her research focuses on wellbeing in higher education. She has 16 years of international and interdisciplinary experience in policy, educational practice, and intervention research.

Seaneen Sloan (Ph.D.) is an associate professor in Education at University College Dublin, Deputy Head of the School of Education, Director of the UCD Centre for the Advancement of Wellbeing, and GUIDE Co-Director. She has over 20 years' experience in academic research and has led and supported over 25 research projects on child and youth wellbeing, including longitudinal cohort studies, randomized controlled trials, qualitative and mixed methods studies, and systematic reviews.

Laura K. Taylor (Ph.D.) is a professor in the School of Psychology at University College Dublin. Her research explores the effects of conflict on children's and adolescents' behaviors, including aggression, prosocial actions, and social identity. With more than 20 years of experience in academia and the public sector, she has published more than 110 peer-reviewed works.

Chapter 2
Ethical Considerations for Cross-National, Longitudinal Research with Children and Families

Stephanie Cahill

Introduction

Growing Up in Digital Europe (GUIDE) is Europe's first comparative cohort study of child and youth wellbeing (see Chap. 1 in this book). This large-scale initiative tracks children from birth to young adulthood, gathering harmonized data across family, school, and community contexts to generate high-quality evidence that can inform policies addressing social, developmental, and health inequalities across Europe (see Chap. 9 in this book). However, conducting ethically sound research with children and families in a multinational, multilingual, and multiregional context introduces considerable challenges.

Significant ethical dilemmas arise from diverse national interpretations of childhood, shaped by social, cultural, and legal norms (Oates, 2020). For instance, Scandinavian countries prioritize children's agency in decision-making, while others, such as Slovenia, uphold more traditional parental authority. Such differences influence children's participation and the implementation of ethical processes such as informed consent. Additionally, managing compliance with legal frameworks such as GDPR adds further complexity, especially when collecting sensitive health or biometric data. Researchers must navigate these legal and cultural nuances to ensure the study is conducted lawfully, respectfully, and with cultural sensitivity in every location.

GUIDE's ethical approach adapts established principles to its specific context. Internationally, human-subject research ethics are grounded in frameworks such as the Declaration of Helsinki (World Medical Association, 2013), the Belmont Report (National Commission for the Protection of Human Subjects of Biomedical & Behavioral Research, 1979), and child-specific rights instruments such as

S. Cahill (✉)
Manchester Institute of Education, University of Manchester, Manchester, England
e-mail: stephanie.cahill@manchester.ac.uk

Policy, Evaluation and Research Unit, Manchester Metropolitan University, Manchester, UK

L. K. Taylor et al. (eds.), *Growing Up in Digital Europe*, Springer Series on Child and Family Studies, https://doi.org/10.1007/978-3-032-30592-3_2

the United Nations Convention on the Rights of the Child (UNCRC; adopted by the United Nations General Assembly, 1989). While these frameworks provide a fundamental baseline, formal guidelines alone do not guarantee ethical practice in real-world settings. Indeed, standardized procedures often fall short when researchers encounter unanticipated dilemmas in the field (Kousholt & Juhl, 2023). Contemporary discourse highlights that children must be viewed not just as vulnerable subjects to be protected, but as individuals with rights and agency. An ethical framework must therefore balance protection with participation, upholding children's welfare and privacy while also respecting their voices and developing capacities, all within the constraints of varying regulations and cultural expectations.

This chapter outlines how GUIDE addresses these ethical considerations in a harmonized yet flexible manner. It reviews foundational ethical principles and GDPR management in a cross-national study, then examines the social constructions of childhood to illustrate the need for culturally sensitive protocols. Subsequent sections focus on practical implementation: obtaining age-appropriate informed consent and assent, safeguarding data privacy (especially sensitive and digital data), and ensuring inclusivity. Finally, it anticipates future challenges, from the rise of new technologies and online research tools to potential expansion into biological data, and considers strategies for "future-proofing" the ethical framework. By establishing shared protocols that allow local adaptation, GUIDE aims to conduct research that is scientifically robust, culturally respectful, and uniformly ethical across Europe.

Foundational Ethical Principles and Guidelines

Research involving children across nations must be grounded in established ethical frameworks that safeguard human subjects. Three cornerstone documents inform current best practices: the Declaration of Helsinki, the Belmont Report, and the UN Convention on the Rights of the Child (UNCRC).

The Declaration of Helsinki, first established in 1964, sets fundamental principles for ethical medical research, emphasizing participant wellbeing, informed consent, and special protections for vulnerable groups (World Medical Association, 2013). Crucially, it mandates that the interests of the research subject must prevail over the interests of science. This is vital when working with children who cannot fully advocate for themselves. The Belmont Report (1979) further outlines three fundamental ethical principles: Respect for Persons, which recognizes individual autonomy and requires informed consent, with additional safeguards for those with diminished autonomy, such as children (requiring parental consent and child assent); Beneficence, which requires maximizing benefits and minimizing harms to participants, aligning with the duty of care toward child wellbeing; and Justice, which demands fairness in participant selection and in the distribution of research burdens and benefits, preventing exploitation or unwarranted exclusion of any group of children or families. Together, Helsinki and Belmont provide an ethical foundation that underpins institutional review board standards worldwide.

Complementing these, the UNCRC (1989) introduced a rights-based framework specific to minors, asserting that children are holders of human rights and active social actors, not merely passive recipients of protection. It enshrines principles such as the best interests of the child (Article 3) and the right of the child to be heard in matters affecting them (Article 12). This challenges paternalistic views and requires investigators to seek ways to inform and involve children appropriately in decisions, consistent with their evolving capacities.

While frameworks such as Helsinki, Belmont, and the UNCRC provide universal principles, their implementation regarding autonomy and informed consent varies significantly by culture and legal context. All European countries, for example, have ratified the UNCRC, committing to its standards for children's rights, yet conceptions of autonomy or informed consent can differ. Harmonizing ethics across multiple countries is a key challenge, often requiring common protocols that meet the highest standard required by any country's regulations.

One practical strategy is creating an international ethics advisory board or working group. For instance, the multi-country Human Early-Life Exposome (HELIX) study created an ethics task force that developed unified guidance on privacy, consent, and data protection for all partner sites (Maitre et al., 2018). This approach fosters consistency while respecting local diversity. Ultimately, these foundational frameworks serve as a common language that must be translated into context-specific practice in each nation, ensuring ethics equivalence across the entire project.

A particularly complex arena for cross-national studies is data protection, which was substantially tightened by the introduction of the EU's General Data Protection Regulation (GDPR) in 2018 (Voigt & Von dem Bussche, 2017), with the UK retaining a domestic version post-Brexit. GDPR is now the baseline, requiring stringent safeguards for processing personal data, with specific additional protection for children's data (Voigt & Von dem Bussche, 2017). Recital 38 explicitly notes that children merit specific protection because they are less aware of risks and consequences regarding their personal information. In practice, longitudinal studies must implement strong data security (e.g., encryption), clear data minimization, and transparency. Consent documentation must be GDPR-compliant and written in language children and parents can understand. Participants also have enforceable rights, such as the right to access their data or the right to be forgotten, which research teams must accommodate (see Chap. 8 in this book).

Cross-national projects also face hurdles such as national variations in the "digital age of consent" and restrictions on cross-border transfers of personal data outside the EU/EEA (see Box 2.1). The LifeCycle Project effectively adapted to these constraints by employing a federated data model, choosing not to centralize identifiable data but instead to conduct analyses within each country's secure system and share only aggregate results (Jaddoe et al., 2020; see Table 2.1 for more information). This demonstrates how multi-country studies can remain collaborative and compliant.

In summary, foundational principles and modern regulations together mandate that multi-country child research be conducted with rigorous consent processes, privacy protections, and a commitment to children's rights.

Table 2.1 Information about Previous Cohort Studies

Study Name	Focus	Key Ethical Practices	Relevance to GUIDE	Citation
Toronto Adolescent and Youth Cohort Study	Neuroimaging and biosample collection among adolescents	Tailored informed consent, inclusion strategies for underrepresented groups, and enhanced data privacy measures	Demonstrates adaptive consent processes and handling of sensitive biomarkers, relevant for GUIDE's future biomarker data collection	Dickie et al. (2024)
Healthy Brain and Child Development Study	Biospecimen collection among underrepresented American Indian communities	Culturally sensitive consent, community consultation, integration of traditional knowledge	Offers insights into engaging diverse communities, important for GUIDE's multinational scope	Bakhireva et al. (2020)
LifeCycle Project – EU Child Cohort Network	Harmonization of data across European cohorts	Federated data infrastructure, transparent governance for ethical data use	Provides a model for cross-national data integration, aligning with GUIDE's aim for harmonized datasets	Jaddoe et al. (2020)
HELIX Study	Early-life environmental exposures and child health	Ethics Task Force guidance, protocols for privacy and data protection	Highlights governance structures for ethical biomarker use, applicable to GUIDE's multi-cohort design	Maitre et al. (2018)
ALSPAC	Linkage of participants to external datasets (e.g., CLA and CIN Census)	Strategies to enhance inclusivity and address attrition in vulnerable families	Informs GUIDE's retention strategies, particularly for underrepresented groups	Boyd et al. (2013)
Born in Bradford	Trust-building fieldwork with marginalized groups (e.g., the Roma community)	Community engagement for better representation and data quality	Highlights the importance of local community relationships in GUIDE's data collection efforts	Born in Bradford (2023), Wright et al. (2013)

(continued)

Table 2.1 (continued)

Study Name	Focus	Key Ethical Practices	Relevance to GUIDE	Citation
UKHLS	Inclusive sampling with ethnic boost samples and tracking fostered children	Innovative approaches to capturing transient populations	Suggests strategies for GUIDE to include and analyze vulnerable populations	University of Essex, Institute for Social and Economic Research (2024)
SEED	Socio-economic stratification via child benefits records	Enhanced precision in sampling and increased heterogeneity	Offers GUIDE a framework for efficient, targeted sampling strategies	Morris et al. (2017)

Box 2.1 Variation in Digital Age of Consent across EU

Under GDPR Article 8, member states can set the 'digital age of consent' between 13 and 16 (default 16). This creates a patchwork of ages: the UK, Sweden, Denmark, and Portugal use 13; Spain uses 14; Slovenia and France require 15; and Germany, Ireland, and Croatia retain 16.

These differences require researchers to tailor consent strategies. For instance, an online survey for a 14-year-old requires parental consent in Germany (age 16) but not in the UK (age 13). To ensure universal compliance, many cross-national studies adopt the most conservative approach (seeking parental consent up to age 16). While this can complicate recruitment, it avoids legal and ethical pitfalls.

Social Constructions of Childhood and Cultural Sensitivity

Ethical research with children must account for the fact that childhood is a social and cultural construct, not a uniform experience. Conceptions of a "child's" role, dependence, and innocence vary widely, impacting research design (James & Prout, 2003). These differences have significant implications for longitudinal studies and require a culturally sensitive approach. Sociological and anthropological perspectives emphasize that features often seen as "natural" childhood traits (such as dependence or innocence) are socially produced, influencing how children are viewed and treated (James et al., 1998). Historically, many Western societies characterized children as vulnerable, passive, and in need of protection and guidance. This view, sometimes termed the deficit model of childhood, treated children as "adults in the making," not yet competent, not yet responsible, effectively disempowering them in research contexts (Carter, 2009). Research practices mirrored these assumptions, with children often positioned as *objects* of study rather than active contributors and adults (researchers, parents) firmly in control of decision-making. For example, until recent decades it was common for research ethics committees to waive the requirement to seek children's assent on the grounds that only parental permission mattered; this reflected a cultural construction of children as lacking agency (Alderson & Morrow, 2020).

Contemporary understandings, influenced by the UNCRC and the "new sociology of childhood," challenge these narratives. The UNCRC's affirmation of children's participatory rights (e.g., the right to express views freely in matters affecting them) has helped recast children as active social actors and experts on their own lives (Oates, 2020). However, this shift is not uniform, as cultural constructions of childhood continue to shape family views on research, consent, and interview techniques (Greene & Stiefvater, 2019; Ortiz-Ospina & Roser, 2016). These constructions influence participation: in communities where children are expected to defer to adults, inviting them to voice opinions may encounter reluctance, whereas in contexts that prize child autonomy, not listening to the child would be unethical. Such differences affect everything from consent processes to interview techniques and data interpretation.

Family roles and decision-making hierarchies add another layer of complexity. In many European contexts, parents act as proxies for their children, whereas in extended-family or collectivist cultures, elders or community leaders may be key decision-makers. Norms about who can provide consent can vary: European and North American norms assume a parent (usually mother or father) gives permission, but elsewhere, a paternal uncle, a grandparent, or another household head may be culturally empowered to speak for the family (Colom & Rohloff, 2018). Researchers should be aware of these dynamics to avoid ethical missteps, engaging community authorities where appropriate and accommodating family decision-making processes, while upholding voluntary and informed participation.

These differences are clear when contrasting European contexts. In Scandinavia, a strong ethos of children's rights supports participatory models where children are sometimes treated as co-researchers, and ethics focus on facilitating genuine participation (Kiili et al., 2025). In contrast, research with some Roma communities in parts of Eastern Europe, where intergenerational hierarchies are strongly upheld and research may be viewed with suspicion due to discrimination (UNICEF, 2007), requires trust-building and engaging community gatekeepers (Condon et al., 2019). Socioeconomic factors, such as economic precarity and limited access to education among Roma families, may further affect feasibility and the perceived value of the research (Kurum Tiryakioglu & Bulbul, 2024; Ringold et al., 2005). Standard questions that assume formal schooling, stable homes, or digital access can inadvertently exclude or stigmatize, requiring adapted methods (e.g., using oral or visual approaches) and ensuring participation does not reinforce existing vulnerabilities (European Union Agency for Fundamental Rights, 2016). Research with marginalized children must go beyond procedural compliance to engage with the structural inequalities affecting their agency and safety. For GUIDE, this means investing in culturally competent fieldworker training, partnering with Roma-led organizations, and co-designing research processes that reflect participant realities (see Chaps. 3, 5, and 9 in this book).

These examples underscore that protocols must be calibrated to the cultural context (Kousholt & Juhl, 2023). This is not cultural relativism; rather, it means finding culturally appropriate ways to honor universal principles such as voluntary and informed participation (Third et al., 2025). This includes recognizing power differentials not only between adults and children but also intra-European hierarchies, such as those between majority populations and historically marginalized communities like the Roma, which shape how research is received, whose voices are valued, and whose interests are prioritized. In summary, recognizing childhood as a social construct confirms that "one-size-fits-all" ethical protocols are inadequate in multinational research.

Informed Consent, Assent, and Data Privacy

Obtaining truly informed consent in cross-national longitudinal studies with children requires age-appropriate, ongoing processes that respect both the child's developing autonomy and the parent or guardian's legal role. Best practices emphasize that children are not merely research subjects but rights-holders whose capacities evolve over time (Maguire et al., 2018). International frameworks and instruments such as the UNCRC stress that children's views be given "due weight" according to age and maturity. Researchers must therefore seek the child's assent and involvement at every stage, even when parental consent is legally mandatory (UK Research & Innovation, 2022), using transparent, child-centered processes, not just procedural forms.

Research with children demands creative strategies to inform and empower young participants. Rather than relying on lengthy paper forms alone, studies now use layered or dynamic consent models that present information in stages or interactive formats (Facca et al., 2020; UK Research & Innovation, 2022). A layered approach might begin with a simple overview and progressively reveal more details, matching the child's capacity and curiosity. For example, information could be provided via multiple child-friendly channels: a newsletter for families, an interactive website about the project, and in-class explanations by teachers (Cowie & Khoo, 2017). Such strategies, coupled with multimedia tools, can significantly improve comprehension and engagement. Digital platforms allow multimodal communication, combining text with videos, animations, or quizzes, to scaffold children's understanding and maintain their interest. Ultimately, the onus is on researchers to employ methods that make consent meaningful, fostering voluntary and positive participation from children (Cowie & Khoo, 2017).

Across jurisdictions, legal requirements differ on when a minor can consent on their own. In most European contexts, a parent or legal guardian's consent is mandatory for participants under 18, but ethical practice goes further to respect the child's wishes. Guidelines in the UK advise that even when children are not legally competent to consent, their assent should be sought whenever practicable, and their dissent respected (UK Research & Innovation, 2022). If a child can understand (often judged on a case-by-case basis, known as "Gillick competence" in British law), researchers should involve them as much as possible in the decision. Indeed, the principle of *evolving capacities* holds that as children grow, they should gain greater autonomy in research participation decisions (Maguire et al., 2018). In practical terms, this means an older adolescent's informed refusal to join a study would override parental wishes, and conversely, ethics committees are increasingly open to a minor's own consent in certain low-risk studies or for those nearing adulthood. Consent is further complicated in separated families: while one parent's consent is often legally sufficient for a child's participation, active objection from another must be resolved (Children Act 1989; General Medical Council, 2018). For GUIDE, this means balancing legal sufficiency with ethical prudence: obtaining consent from one parent may be lawful, but transparent communication and sensitivity to family dynamics are essential.

Application of these principles into practice can vary depending on national law. Some countries legally allow adolescents (16 + or even younger in specific cases) to consent to research or certain treatments, while others require parental consent up to age 18. Researchers must navigate these differences carefully. On one hand, requiring parental permission can become a barrier. Studies on sensitive topics have found that some youths will not participate if they must inform their parents (Hokke et al., 2018). For example, a digital survey of LGBTQ + teens in the US waived parental consent to protect participants who might be put at risk by outing themselves to parents (Hoffman et al., 2009). Additionally, evidence from school-based public health research shows that requiring active parental consent can substantially reduce participation rates and bias samples, under-representing certain groups of young people (Bonell et al., 2023). On the other hand, parental engagement can be positive when approached collaboratively. The key is to balance protection with empowerment: ensure parents or guardians are appropriately involved while continuously affirming the child's right to understand and choose. Cross-national projects such as GUIDE may need flexible consent protocols that adhere to each country's laws but uphold a common ethic of child assent and agency (e.g., providing translated, contextually relevant explanations and obtaining dual parent–child agreement where possible).

Longitudinal research often collects sensitive information, such as health status, psychological assessments, or biological samples (e.g., saliva or blood for biomarkers; see Chap. 7 in this book). Under the GDPR, health and biometric data are classified as special category data, requiring explicit consent and strong protection measures (encryption, restricted access, etc.). Researchers should clearly communicate why these data are needed, how they will be used, and who will have access (see Chap. 8 in this book). An age-appropriate explanation of risks is critical – for instance, explaining what a genetic sample is and ensuring families understand any future implications of its use. Interactive consent tools can help here as well; for example, a tablet-based quiz could check a teenager's understanding of what giving a DNA sample entails and allow questions in real time. Moreover, ethics protocols should address incidental findings (like an unexpected health issue revealed by a biomarker) and how results will be communicated to parents or participants, all while prioritizing the child's welfare.

A recent review noted the challenge of verifying parental consent online. Some minors might attempt to fraudulently complete a parent's consent form, so one study confirmed consent by following up via phone and asking parents basic questions about the study to confirm their awareness (Hokke et al., 2018). Such diligence helps ensure that consent is genuine and informed. Beyond the initial consent process, studies must also address how data are governed and protected once collected. In line with GDPR principles, data minimization and robust anonymization or pseudonymization of child data are crucial. Many large EU cohort projects now use privacy-by-design approaches. This kind of governance, with clear data sharing agreements and oversight, upholds participants' privacy across nations.

Equally important are participants' enforceable rights under GDPR: children (and their parents or guardians) have the right to access their data, withdraw consent, or request deletion. To respect these rights, studies must establish transparent communication plans and accessible mechanisms throughout the study, ensuring families understand how they can exercise control over their information (see Chap. 8 in this book).

In long-term research, consent is not a one-off event but an active, continuous process. Children's circumstances and understanding can change significantly over the years of a longitudinal study. Ethical studies therefore implement re-consent or assent renewal at key intervals. For example, a child enrolled at birth should be re-informed and asked for their own consent or assent at a later age when capable of understanding the study, rather than relying solely on the parental consent given years earlier. It is good practice to "check in" at each new wave to confirm that the child and the parent are still willing to continue. This might involve sending updated information sheets or engaging participants with new multimedia summaries of the project's progress and any new procedures.

In recent years, some longitudinal projects have used digital tools within the consent process. Dynamic consent platforms, secure online portals or apps, allow participants (and parents) to review how their data are being used, update contact preferences, and even consent to optional new sub-studies (Wallace & Miola, 2021). Such tools treat consent as "provisional, ongoing and dependent on relationships," maintaining dialogue and trust between researchers and participants (Wallace & Miola, 2021). A participatory research project in New Zealand, for instance, found it effective to negotiate consent continually with youth co-researchers over an 18-month period, rather than assuming that a one-time form was sufficient (Loveridge et al., 2024). The researcher stayed attentive to "youth cues" and regularly reaffirmed each young person's willingness to engage, highlighting how ongoing consent can be woven into research interactions. This dynamic approach is particularly important when new sensitive measures are introduced mid-study (for example, adding a biobank or mental health module in a later wave); participants should have the opportunity to opt in or out at that point, even if they agreed to earlier components. By treating consent as a process of dialogue rather than a bureaucratic hurdle, longitudinal studies can adapt to children's growing autonomy while continually safeguarding their welfare and privacy (Facca et al., 2020).

Inclusivity and Representation

Ensuring inclusivity is both an ethical and methodological imperative. Without deliberate strategies to engage marginalized populations (e.g., those in poverty, ethnic minorities, or migrant families), large-scale cohorts risk reinforcing inequality by generating knowledge that only reflects privileged groups.

Several large-scale studies have shown that inclusivity cannot be left to chance but must be embedded structurally in study design. For example, the Born in Bradford (BiB) cohort invested in long-term relationships with local community organizations and community leaders, employing bilingual fieldworkers and culturally sensitive approaches to engage diverse minority populations, particularly families of Pakistani heritage, who make up a large proportion of the Bradford community (Wright et al., 2013; see Table 2.1 for more information). In other European contexts, research engaging Gypsy, Roma, and Traveler communities highlights the need for trust-building and tailored methods to overcome barriers of exclusion and mistrust (Condon et al., 2019; UNICEF, 2007). For instance, Understanding Society (UKHLS) used an Ethnic Minority Boost Sample (EMBS) at Wave 1, later supplemented by an Immigrant and Ethnic Minority Boost (IEMBS) at Wave 6 (University of Essex, Institute for Social and Economic Research, 2024; see Table 2.1 for more information). Furthermore, its household-based longitudinal design enables continued inclusion of children even as they move between households, contributing to ethical retention of participants in transient circumstances, such as foster children (Institute for Social and Economic Research, 2021). These examples illustrate the principle that inclusive recruitment requires not only methodological adaptation but also cultural competence and engagement with local communities. The ethical rationale for these strategies is clear: participation should not exacerbate existing vulnerabilities or reproduce systemic exclusion. For GUIDE, inclusivity means going beyond statistical representativeness to ensure that children from disadvantaged or marginalized backgrounds have equal opportunities to contribute to, and benefit from, research evidence. As noted in studies such as ALSPAC, attrition is highest among families with socioeconomic disadvantage, meaning that without sustained engagement and tailored retention strategies, longitudinal cohorts risk systematically losing the very voices most needed to inform policy on inequality (Boyd et al., 2013; see Table 2.1 for more information).

The increasing reliance on digital tools for recruitment and consent presents both opportunities/flexibility and risks regarding inclusivity. Data from the EU's *State of the Digital Decade* (European Commission, 2024) shows that only about 55.6% of adult Europeans currently possess basic digital skills, with deficits most pronounced among those with lower education, manual occupations, or rural residency. Thus, digital tools can create new barriers for families with limited digital access or literacy. These risks amplify social exclusion, with families in poverty or recent migrant groups disproportionately disadvantaged (Hokke et al., 2018). GUIDE's ethical protocols should therefore include accessible, non-digital alternatives (e.g., plain language materials, in-person support) to ensure equitable participation. Moreover, "layered consent" models should be applied to mitigate comprehension barriers for both parents and children (Facca et al., 2020).

Researchers face a persistent dilemma in practical feasibility with the moral obligation not to exclude vulnerable groups. Selective exclusion often arises under the guise of methodological purity: for instance, excluding children in foster care, those with disabilities, or those living in non-traditional households on the grounds of data comparability. Yet such exclusions risk producing evidence that is systematically biased against those most affected by structural disadvantages. The SEED study demonstrated that linking recruitment to administrative data sources, such as child benefit records, enabled inclusion of families from diverse socioeconomic backgrounds who would otherwise have been missed (Morris et al., 2017; see Table 2.1 for more information). Similarly, GUIDE should advocate for harmonized inclusion standards to avoid reinforcing hierarchies of whose childhoods "count" in European data (see Chaps. 4 and 9 in this book).

Compensation also intersects with inclusivity. While some jurisdictions permit only token payments for children's participation, others allow more substantial forms of reimbursement or recognition (Nuffield Council on Bioethics, 2015). Fair reimbursement for costs and time can reduce participation barriers for low-SES families, particularly by offsetting travel and childcare costs (Bonevski et al., 2014). The ethical principle here is twofold: first, children and families should not be left worse off by participating in research; second, payments should not be so large as to unduly influence consent. The ethical approach is to standardize principles (e.g., cover all costs, be proportionate to time) rather than specific amounts, ensuring payments are non-coercive and culturally respectful. Guidance from the Ethical Research Involving Children (ERIC) project recommends distinguishing between reimbursement for direct expenses, recognition of time and effort, and incentives, with each handled transparently and proportionately (Graham et al., 2013). A balanced approach for GUIDE is therefore to standardize principles rather than specific amounts: for example, compensation should cover legitimate costs, be proportionate to time and effort, and be structured in ways that avoid stigma or inequity, such as vouchers usable in multiple settings where cash raises concerns. Importantly, involving children and families in shaping what forms of compensation feel appropriate can further enhance fairness and trust, ensuring that practices are not only legally compliant but also culturally respectful and ethically robust across all participating countries (see Chap. 4 in this book).

Taken together, inclusivity is central to GUIDE's ethical legitimacy. By embedding inclusive recruitment, addressing digital inequities, and adopting fair compensation, GUIDE can position itself as a model of equitable cohort research. Moreover, these practices will enhance the validity and policy relevance of findings across diverse European populations.

Future-Proofing Ethical Frameworks

Longitudinal studies such as GUIDE are, by definition, designed to extend over decades, following children as they grow into adulthood and, in some cases, into the next generation. This temporal scale presents unique ethical challenges, as decisions must anticipate unforeseen legal, technological, and social changes. To remain credible and legitimate, GUIDE's ethical framework must be adaptive, responding to new developments while maintaining the trust that long-term participation requires (see Box 2.2).

A major driver of change is technological innovation. The increasing use of digital trace data, wearable devices, and passive sensing tools raises new ethical dilemmas about privacy, surveillance, and consent. Wearable sensors, for example, may reveal sensitive information about children's movements or health that was not envisaged when families first consented. Research has highlighted how consumer wearables, though attractive for their low cost and accessibility, introduce complex ethical risks relating to data sharing and participant awareness (Canali et al., 2023; Sui et al., 2023). Artificial intelligence and machine learning techniques, now integral to analyzing complex datasets, also bring risks of algorithmic bias and opacity. GUIDE must build in mechanisms to regularly review and update its data governance policies to protect participant rights as methodologies evolve.

The evolution of legal frameworks, such as the GDPR, also shapes the ethical landscape. Future regulations on AI or cross-border data flows will require further adaptation. GUIDE must anticipate these changes with flexible governance. Work on large-scale European pilots such as GATEKEEPER illustrates the complexity of navigating national variations in ethical and legal approvals, underlining the need for harmonized but adaptable governance models (Maccaro et al., 2024). A promising model is the "living" ethical protocol. This protocol is periodically reviewed and revised in consultation with ethics boards, legal experts, and participant advisory groups, an approach that avoids the rigidity of a single framework while ensuring ongoing compliance and responsiveness to change.

Dynamic consent models offer another avenue for future-proofing. Traditional one-time consent is increasingly seen as insufficient for studies that span decades and incorporate new data types over time. Dynamic consent, delivered through digital platforms, enables participants to revisit, reaffirm, or adjust their preferences as circumstances evolve. Longitudinal biobanks such as the CHRIS study in Italy have demonstrated how dynamic consent can promote participant engagement, strengthen communication, and improve long-term sustainability (Mascalzoni et al., 2022). Dynamic consent platforms are becoming increasingly feasible and user-friendly, giving participants a greater sense of agency and control (Teare et al., 2021). While dynamic consent presents challenges in terms of infrastructure, digital access, and potential participant burden, its adoption in GUIDE could serve as a powerful demonstration of ethical innovation in cohort research.

Future-proofing also requires a proactive stance on emerging areas of vulnerability. Climate change, digitalization, and shifting family structures are already transforming children's daily lives, and with them the ethical questions facing researchers. For example, collecting biomarker or genetic data may be scientifically valuable (see Chap. 7 in this book), but raises questions about long-term storage, incidental findings, and the future use of data beyond the original study aims. Similarly, linking cohort data to administrative records on education, health, or social care can improve analytic power but heightens concerns about surveillance, consent, and potential misuse by authorities. GUIDE should remain vigilant to these risks, ensuring that expansions in scope are always accompanied by careful ethical review and renewed engagement with children and families.

Central to future-proofing is the recognition that children themselves will grow into adults and, eventually, parents who may be asked to re-consent on behalf of their own children. GUIDE should plan for this intergenerational transition by embedding mechanisms to refresh consent as participants reach adulthood, and by recognizing the evolving capacities of children as decision-makers. A cohort designed to last decades must treat participants not as static subjects but as partners whose rights and roles change over time.

Finally, GUIDE's ethical resilience depends on continuous dialogue with its stakeholders. Establishing standing ethics advisory boards, including youth representatives, community members, and multi-disciplinary experts, can help ensure that evolving risks and opportunities are identified early. Transparency is key: by communicating openly with participants about how GUIDE adapts to new challenges, the study can maintain the trust that is essential for long-term retention and impact.

Box 2.2 Recommendations for Ethical Adaptation to Emerging Technologies

- Develop "living" ethical protocols, subject to regular review and revision.
- Monitor emerging technologies (AI, wearables, digital trace data) and update governance accordingly.
- Explore dynamic consent platforms to allow participants to revisit or modify choices.
- Ensure flexibility to adapt to evolving legal frameworks across Europe.
- Embed re-consent procedures as children reach adulthood, recognizing evolving capacities.
- Anticipate new ethical challenges in areas such as biomarker collection and administrative data linkage.
- Maintain standing ethics advisory boards, including youth voices, to identify and respond to emerging issues.
- Commit to transparency and regular communication with participants about ethical adaptations.

Conclusion and Recommendations

The establishment of GUIDE represents a landmark opportunity to advance ethical standards in cross-national, longitudinal child research. As a study designed to endure for decades, across multiple countries, generations, and political landscapes, its ethical framework must therefore be both rights-based and flexible to adapting to future changes in law, technology, and society.

This chapter highlighted several core imperatives. First, inclusivity is an ethical requirement: GUIDE must invest in strategies to reach and retain marginalized children and families, ensuring that those whose voices are most often absent in research are central to its evidence base. Second, the framework must be future-oriented. Emerging technologies, dynamic consent models, and evolving legal frameworks will all reshape the ethical terrain. GUIDE must therefore institutionalize review and renewal processes, ensuring that its practices remain aligned with the highest standards of integrity and respect.

Finally, GUIDE's ethical resilience will depend on sustained dialogue with participants themselves, treating them as partners, not just subjects, through mechanisms for reconsent and participatory governance.

GUIDE is uniquely positioned to set a benchmark for ethical cohort research in Europe. By integrating inclusivity, future-proofed governance, and participant-centered approaches, GUIDE can not only maintain trust across generations but also demonstrate how large-scale child research can be both scientifically robust and ethically exemplary.

References

Alderson, P., & Morrow, V. (2020). *The ethics of research with children and young people: A practical handbook* (2nd ed.). Sage. https://doi.org/10.4135/9781529682694

Bakhireva, L. N., Nebeker, C., Ossorio, P., Angal, J., Thomason, M. E., & Croff, J. M. (2020). Inclusion of American Indians and Alaskan Natives in large national studies: Ethical considerations and implications for biospecimen collection in the healthy brain and child development study. *Adversity and Resilience Science, 1*(4), 285–294. https://doi.org/10.1007/s42844-020-00020-8

Bonell, C., Humphrey, N., Singh, I., Viner, R. M., & Ford, T. (2023). Approaches to consent in public health research in secondary schools. *BMJ Open, 13*(6), Article e070277. https://doi.org/10.1136/bmjopen-2022-070277

Bonevski, B., Randell, M., Paul, C., Chapman, K., Twyman, L., Bryant, J., Brozek, I., & Hughes, C. (2014). Reaching the hard-to-reach: A systematic review of strategies for improving health and medical research with socially disadvantaged groups. *BMC Medical Research Methodology, 14*(1), Article 42. https://doi.org/10.1186/1471-2288-14-42

Born in Bradford. (2023). *Evidence briefing—Air quality: Pollution and health.* https://borninbradford.nhs.uk/wp-content/uploads/HG2929-BIHR-BiB-Evidence-Briefing-CAZ-Air-Quality-10.pdf

Boyd, A., Golding, J., Macleod, J., Lawlor, D. A., Fraser, A., Henderson, J., Molloy, L., Ness, A., Ring, S., & Davey Smith, G. (2013). Cohort profile: The 'children of the 90s'—the index offspring of the Avon Longitudinal Study of Parents and Children. *International Journal of Epidemiology, 42*(1), 111–127. https://doi.org/10.1093/ije/dys064

Canali, S., De Marchi, B., & Aliverti, A. (2023). Wearable technologies and stress: Toward an ethically grounded approach. *International Journal of Environmental Research and Public Health, 20*(18), 6737. https://doi.org/10.3390/ijerph20186737

Carter, B. (2009). Tick box for child? The ethical positioning of children as vulnerable, researchers as barbarians and reviewers as overly cautious. *International Journal of Nursing Studies, 46*(6), 858–864. https://doi.org/10.1016/j.ijnurstu.2009.01.003

Children Act. (1989). c. 41. https://www.legislation.gov.uk/ukpga/1989/41/contents

Colom, M., & Rohloff, P. (2018). Cultural considerations for informed consent in paediatric research in low/middle-income countries: A scoping review. *BMJ Paediatrics Open, 2*(1), Article e000298. https://doi.org/10.1136/bmjpo-2018-000298

European Commission. (2024). *State of the digital decade 2024*. https://digital-strategy.ec.europa.eu/en/library/report-state-digital-decade-2024

Condon, L., Bedford, H., Ireland, L., Kerr, S., Mytton, J., Richardson, Z., & Jackson, C. (2019). Engaging Gypsy, Roma, and traveller communities in research: Maximizing opportunities and overcoming challenges. *Qualitative Health Research, 29*(9), 1324–1333. https://doi.org/10.1177/1049732318813558

Cowie, B., & Khoo, E. (2017). Accountability through access, authenticity and advocacy when researching with young children. *International Journal of Inclusive Education, 21*(3), 234–247. https://doi.org/10.1080/13603116.2016.1260821

Dickie, E. W., Ameis, S. H., Boileau, I., Diaconescu, A. O., Felsky, D., Goldstein, B. I., Gonçalves, V., Griffiths, J. D., Haltigan, J. D., & Husain, M. O. (2024). Neuroimaging and biosample collection in the Toronto adolescent and youth cohort study: Rationale, methods, and early data. *Biological Psychiatry: Cognitive Neuroscience and Neuroimaging, 9*(3), 275–284. https://doi.org/10.1016/j.bpsc.2023.10.013

European Union Agency for Fundamental Rights. (2016). *Second European Union minorities and discrimination survey: Roma—Selected findings*. Publications Office of the European Union. https://fra.europa.eu/en/publication/2016/second-european-union-minorities-and-discrimination-survey-roma-selected-findings

Facca, D., Smith, M. J., Shelley, J., Lizotte, D., & Donelle, L. (2020). Exploring the ethical issues in research using digital data collection strategies with minors: A scoping review. *PLOS ONE, 15*(8), Article e0237875. https://doi.org/10.1371/journal.pone.0237875

General Medical Council. (2018). *0–18 years: Guidance for all doctors*. https://www.gmc-uk.org/professional-standards/the-professional-standards/0-18-years

Graham, A., Powell, M. A., Taylor, N., Anderson, D., & Fitzgerald, R. (2013). *Ethical research involving children*. UNICEF Office of Research–Innocenti. https://www.unicef.org/innocenti/media/9181/file/Ethical-Research-Involving-Children-compendium-2013-EN.pdf.pdf

Greene, M. E., & Stiefvater, E. (2019). *Social and gender norms and child marriage: A reflection on issues, evidence and areas of inquiry in the field*. ALIGN. https://www.alignplatform.org/resources/2019/04/social-gender-norms-and-child-marriage

Hoffman, N. D., Freeman, K., & Swann, S. (2009). Healthcare preferences of lesbian, gay, bisexual, transgender and questioning youth. *Journal of Adolescent Health, 45*(3), 222–229. https://doi.org/10.1016/j.jadohealth.2009.01.009

Hokke, S., Hackworth, N. J., Quin, N., Bennetts, S. K., Win, H. Y., Nicholson, J. M., Zion, L., Lucke, J., Keyzer, P., & Crawford, S. B. (2018). Ethical issues in using the internet to engage participants in family and child research: A scoping review. *PLOS ONE, 13*(9), Article e0204572. https://doi.org/10.1371/journal.pone.0204572

Institute for Social and Economic Research. (2021, October 30). *Understanding society: Waves 1–11, 2009–2020 and harmonised BHPS: Waves 1–18, 1991–2009, user guide*. https://doc.ukdataservice.ac.uk/doc/6614/mrdoc/pdf/6614_main_survey_user_guide.pdf

Jaddoe, V. W. V., Felix, J. F., Andersen, A.-M.N., Charles, M.-A., Chatzi, L., Corpeleijn, E., Donner, N., Elhakeem, A., Eriksson, J. G., & Foong, R. (2020). The lifecycle project-EU child cohort network: A federated analysis infrastructure and harmonized data of more than 250,000 children and parents. *European Journal of Epidemiology, 35*(7), 709–724. https://doi.org/10.1007/s10654-020-00662-z

James, A., Jenks, C., & Prout, A. (1998). *Theorizing childhood*. Polity Press.

James, A., & Prout, A. (2003). *Constructing and reconstructing childhood: Contemporary issues in the sociological study of childhood*. Routledge.

Kiili, J., Tiina, L.-L., Johanna, M., Sirpa, K., & Malinen, K. (2025). Collaborating with children: Intergenerational research encounters. *International Journal of Social Research Methodology, 28*(1), 105–118. https://doi.org/10.1080/13645579.2024.2301848

Kousholt, D., & Juhl, P. (2023). Addressing ethical dilemmas in research with young children and families: Situated ethics in collaborative research. *Human Arenas, 6*(3), 560–579. https://doi.org/10.1007/s42087-021-00236-9

Kurum Tiryakioglu, G., & Bulbul, T. (2024). Roma children's access to education: Barriers and supports. *Journal of Poverty*, 1–24. https://doi.org/10.1080/10875549.2024.2401348

Loveridge, J., Wood, B. E., Davis-Rae, E., & McRae, H. (2024). Ethical challenges in participatory research with children and youth. *Qualitative Research, 24*(2), 391–411. https://doi.org/10.1177/14687941221149594

Maccaro, A., Tsiompanidou, V., Piaggio, D., Gallego Montejo, A. M., Cea Sánchez, G., de Batlle, J., Quesada Rodriguez, A., Fico, G., & Pecchia, L. (2024). Towards a common European ethical and legal framework for conducting clinical research: The gatekeeper experience. *npj Digital Medicine, 7*(1), 95. https://doi.org/10.1038/s41746-024-01092-x

Maguire, L. K., Byrne, B., & Kehoe, S. (2018). Respecting and fulfilling the right of post-primary pupils to consent to participate in trials and evaluative research: A discussion paper. *International Journal of Research & Method in Education, 41*(1), 89–103. https://doi.org/10.1080/1743727X.2016.1200028

Maitre, L., De Bont, J., Casas, M., Robinson, O., Aasvang, G. M., Agier, L., Andrušaitytė, S., Ballester, F., Basagaña, X., & Borràs, E. (2018). Human Early Life Exposome (HELIX) study: A European population-based exposome cohort. *BMJ Open, 8*(9), Article e021311. https://doi.org/10.1136/bmjopen-2017-021311

Mascalzoni, D., Melotti, R., Pattaro, C., Pramstaller, P. P., Gögele, M., De Grandi, A., & Biasiotto, R. (2022). Ten years of dynamic consent in the CHRIS study: Informed consent as a dynamic process. *European Journal of Human Genetics, 30*(12), 1391–1397. https://doi.org/10.1038/s41431-022-01160-4

Morris, S., Melhuish, E., & Gardiner, J. (2017). *Study of Early Education and Development (SEED): Impact study on early education use and child outcomes up to age three*. Department for Education. https://assets.publishing.service.gov.uk/media/61964d19e90e0704478a9c75/SEED-Age_3_RESEARCH_REPORT.pdf

Nuffield Council on Bioethics. (2015). *Children and clinical research: Ethical issues*. https://www.nuffieldbioethics.org/publication/children-and-clinical-research-ethical-issues/

Oates, J. (2020). Research ethics, children, and young people. In R. Iphofen (Ed.), *Handbook of research ethics and scientific integrity* (pp. 623–635). Springer. https://doi.org/10.1007/978-3-030-16759-2_28

Ortiz-Ospina, E., & Roser, M. (2016). *Child labor*. Our World in Data.

National Commission for the Protection of Human Subjects of Biomedical and Behavioral Research. (1979). *The Belmont report: Ethical principles and guidelines for the protection of human subjects of research* (Vol. 2). Department of Health, Education, and Welfare. https://www.hhs.gov/ohrp/sites/default/files/the-belmont-report-508c_FINAL.pdf

Ringold, D., Orenstein, M. A., & Wilkens, E. (2005). *Roma in an expanding Europe: Breaking the poverty cycle*. World Bank Publications.

Sui, A., Sui, W., Liu, S., & Rhodes, R. (2023). Ethical considerations for the use of consumer wearables in health research. *Digital Health, 9*, 20552076231153740.

Teare, H. J. A., Prictor, M., & Kaye, J. (2021). Reflections on dynamic consent in biomedical research: The story so far. *European Journal of Human Genetics, 29*(4), 649–656. https://doi.org/10.1038/s41431-020-00771-z

Third, A., Baú, V., Tasker, S., & Welland, L. (2025). *Involving children in research and data collection: A gap analysis.* Save the Children International. https://resourcecentre.savethechildren.net/pdf/FINAL_Gap-Analysis-research-brief_25.03.2025.pdf/

UK Research and Innovation. (2022). *MRC/ESRC joint guidance on involving children in research.* https://www.ukri.org/wp-content/uploads/2022/03/MRC-010322-MRCESRCJointGuidanceInvolvingChildrenResearch.pdf

United Nations General Assembly. (1989). Convention on the rights of the child. *United Nations Treaty Series, 1577*(3), 1–23. https://treaties.un.org/pages/ViewDetails.aspx?chapter=4&mtdsg_no=IV-11&src=IND

UNICEF. (2007). *Breaking the cycle of exclusion: Roma children in South East Europe.* https://www.unicef.org/serbia/media/7516/file/Breaking%20the%20cycle%20of%20exclusion.pdf

University of Essex, Institute for Social and Economic Research. (2024). *Understanding society: Waves 1–14, 2009–2023 and harmonised BHPS: Waves 1–18, 1991–2009* (19th ed.). [Data collection]. https://doi.org/10.5255/UKDA-SN-6614-20

Voigt, P., & von dem Bussche, A. (2017). *The EU General Data Protection Regulation (GDPR): A practical guide* (1st ed.). Springer International Publishing.

Wallace, S. E., & Miola, J. (2021). Adding dynamic consent to a longitudinal cohort study: A qualitative study of exceed participant perspectives. *BMC Medical Ethics, 22*(1), 12. https://doi.org/10.1186/s12910-021-00583-w

World Medical Association. (2013). World medical association declaration of Helsinki: Ethical principles for medical research involving human subjects. *JAMA, 310*(20), 2191–2194. https://doi.org/10.1001/jama.2013.281053

Wright, J., Small, N., Raynor, P., Tuffnell, D., Bhopal, R., Cameron, N., Fairley, L., Lawlor, D. A., Parslow, R., & Petherick, E. S. (2013). Cohort profile: The born in Bradford multi-ethnic family cohort study. *International Journal of Epidemiology, 42*(4), 978–991. https://doi.org/10.1093/ije/dys112

Stephanie Cahill (Ph.D.) is a research associate at Manchester Metropolitan University, specializing in child and adolescent wellbeing, life course perspectives, and resilience. Her current research explores children's digital wellbeing, the impact of climate change on mental health, and ethical considerations in research involving children and young people.

Chapter 3
Managing Fieldwork across Contexts: Modes and Methods for Studying Child Wellbeing

Katja Upadyaya, Arttu Brax, and Stephanie Cahill

Managing Fieldwork across Contexts: Modes and Methods for Studying Child Wellbeing

This chapter focuses on GUIDE's fieldwork modes and methods. It presents key aspects of GUIDE's child-centered approach to research design and data collection, including how different fieldwork methods are adapted to engage children in a valuable way. The following sections focus on strategies, logistics, and methods for effective large-scale data collection in social and longitudinal research. It contrasts centralized approaches to data collection—valued for consistency, standardization, and cost efficiency—with decentralized models that offer flexibility and local adaptability, noting that a balanced approach can optimize both quality and efficiency. Building on this, fieldwork logistics are addressed including planning, coordination, adaptation to cultural and geographic contexts, and resource management to ensure smooth operations and high-quality data. Finally, a range of data collection methods are introduced, from web-based and mobile technologies to telephone, online video, and in-person interviews, highlighting their benefits, limitations, and situational uses (Dangubic & Voorpostel, 2017). Case studies from large European panel studies illustrate these concepts and inform GUIDE's first Wave, for a child-centered, cost-effective approach. Furthermore, the chapter also considers the impact of digital transformation over the last 25 years on fieldwork practices, such as the use of digital tools and online platforms for data gathering and interaction with children. The chapter concludes by emphasizing the need for context-specific, culturally

K. Upadyaya (✉) · A. Brax
Department of Education, University of Helsinki, Helsinki, Finland
e-mail: katja.upadyaya@helsinki.fi

S. Cahill
Manchester Institute of Education, University of Manchester, England, UK

L. K. Taylor et al. (eds.), *Growing Up in Digital Europe*, Springer Series on Child and Family Studies, https://doi.org/10.1007/978-3-032-30592-3_3

sensitive methodologies and looking ahead to trends such as digitalization, hybrid modes, and the ethical use of emerging technologies.

Importance of Effective Data Collection in Research

Effective data collection is essential in research as it ensures that the data gathered is relevant, valid, reliable, and accurately aligned with research objectives. Proper data collection methods improve data quality by reducing biases and enhancing accuracy, which are critical for achieving a representative sample and ensuring the credibility and generalizability of findings (see Chap. 9 in this book; Broekstra et al., 2020). Research reliability entails consistency of results over time, while validity refers to the accuracy and truthfulness of what is being measured; both are foundational for producing trustworthy and replicable research outcomes (Babarović et al., 2025; Leung, 2015). Effective data management—such as well-designed data collection tools and clear protocols—helps to minimize errors and preserve research integrity, enabling valid conclusions that can inform policy and advance knowledge across various disciplines (Babarović et al., 2025).

Fieldwork Management

Large-scale fieldwork data collection in social and longitudinal research is largely managed in two ways: centralized or decentralized.

Centralized approaches to data collection involve consolidating data management and decision-making within a single, central authority or team. This approach is characterized by having a unified data platform or repository where data from various sources or units is standardized, integrated, and stored in one place, ensuring consistency and a "single source of truth" across the organization or project. In addition, centralized approaches often feature standardized protocols, streamlined governance, improved security controls, and easier enforcement of data access policies. Such approaches typically facilitate better data quality management, avoid data redundancy, and enable consistent reporting and compliance.

Advantages of centralized approaches include enhanced data integrity and consistency since all users access the same unified dataset; simplified governance and security management due to centralized control; cost efficiency from reduced data duplication and infrastructure savings; and improved analytics and decision-making through comprehensive data integration (Islam & Apu, 2024). However, disadvantages include reduced flexibility and slower responsiveness for individual teams needing tailored data solutions; potential bottlenecks due to reliance on the central team for changes or approvals; risk of creating a one-size-fits-all system that may not meet all local or department-specific needs; and possible challenges accommodating diverse or rapidly evolving requirements.

Large-scale study projects such as the Global Enteric Multicenter Study (GEMS) have utilized centralized data management approaches to ensure consistency, quality, and security across geographically diverse sites. In GEMS, a centralized data coordinating center oversaw the establishment of a centralized database that integrated standardized case report forms, quality control protocols, and a secure transfer system to process more than 1.5 million pages of study data across seven countries (Biswas et al., 2012).

Decentralized approaches to data collection, in turn, involve distributing data management and decision-making responsibilities across multiple local teams, units, or regions rather than centralizing them under a single authority (Islam & Apu, 2024). This approach is characterized by allowing localized control over the design, implementation, and governance of data processes, enabling teams to tailor methods and tools to their specific contexts and needs. In GUIDE, an example would be national teams designing country-specific response options for the surveys (e.g., sources of income which may vary across countries; Babarović et al., 2025). Decentralized systems often feature diverse platforms or repositories managed independently but coordinated through overarching guidelines to maintain a degree of consistency.

Advantages of decentralized approaches include increased flexibility and responsiveness to local conditions, cultural differences, and operational realities. They promote autonomy and innovation at the local level, potentially improving participant engagement and data relevance (Cummins et al., 2023). Decentralized models can reduce bottlenecks associated with central approval processes and allow for quicker adaptation to changing circumstances. Disadvantages include the risk of inconsistent data standards and quality across units, potential duplication of effort and resources, and challenges in enforcing uniform data security and compliance policies. Coordination and integration can become more complex, requiring additional mechanisms to align practices and consolidate data for analysis. In summary, decentralized approaches offer enhanced local adaptability but face challenges maintaining consistent data quality and efficient resource use.

Hanke et al. (2021) outlined how decentralized systems leverage interoperable components to ensure portability, version control, and long-term accessibility of research outputs. By applying a uniform yet flexible data structure, decentralized research data management facilitated data sharing and collaboration across multiple scales. Case studies including the OpenNeuro repository and the Canadian Open Neuroscience Platform demonstrate that decentralization improves inclusivity, mitigates risks associated with centralized failures, and allows institutions to retain governance over their data while still enabling interoperability (Hanke et al., 2021).

Fieldwork Management Approaches and Efficiency in Managing Data and Resources

When comparing centralized and decentralized approaches in terms of efficiency, the key distinction lies in how each model balances control, standardization, and resource optimization against flexibility, adaptability, and local autonomy. In Table 3.1, centralized and decentralized approaches are compared further (see also Briceno-Rosas et al., 2020; Khalilov, 2023).

In practice, many research projects, such as GUIDE, adopt a hybrid approach, integrating centralized coordination for key governance and quality assurance with decentralized execution for local responsiveness. This combination aims to maximize efficiency by leveraging the strengths of both models: central oversight ensures alignment and quality, while local autonomy maintains flexibility and contextual relevance.

Table 3.1 Centralized and decentralized fieldwork management

	Centralized approach	Decentralized approach
Efficiency in data management	High efficiency through uniform standards, streamlined governance, and reduced duplication of effort. Easier data integration and consistency.	Lower efficiency due to possible duplication of effort, varied data standards, and complexity in integrating data from multiple sources.
Resource utilization	Optimizes use of infrastructure and resources centrally, often leading to lower overall costs.	Resources spread across multiple units, potentially causing redundant efforts and higher costs overall.
Flexibility & Adaptability	Less flexible, slower to adapt to local needs, may create bottlenecks in decision-making.	More flexible and responsive to local conditions and specific needs, allowing tailored solutions.
Control & Standardization	Strong centralized control ensures consistent policies, data quality, and compliance.	Weaker control can lead to inconsistent data quality and compliance challenges.
Scalability	Scalability is limited by central capacity; it can become a bottleneck at large scale.	Generally more scalable by adding local units or nodes.
Management complexity	Easier centralized management, one point of oversight.	More complex due to managing multiple independent units, requiring coordination mechanisms.
Cost implications	Typically lower data management costs as duplicated tasks are minimized.	Generally higher costs due to duplication, additional organizational layers, and less streamlined operations.

Fieldwork Logistics

Planning and Coordination

Fieldwork planning.

in GUIDE is based on national population size: countries with over ten million inhabitants target 10,000 infants and 8000 8-year-olds; smaller countries aim for half these numbers to allow for attrition (see Chap. 4 in this book). The national teams carry out the fieldwork in collaboration with the Central Hub, Centerdata, and survey agencies. National teams and the Central Hub prepare questionnaires and related materials, while agencies secure the technical equipment needed for interviews. Clear timelines, budgets, and role allocation ensure adherence to the GUIDE sampling procedures (Babarović et al., 2025; Upadyaya et al., 2025).

Similar research projects tailor sample sizes according to population characteristics and attrition risks, ensuring robust longitudinal designs. For example, large-scale assessment studies such as PISA use different stratification designs when tailoring sample sizes to guarantee a representative sample of the population (Mang et al., 2024). Coordination with centralized units and local agencies helps balance consistency and local expertise (see also Briceno-Rosas et al., 2020; Khalilov, 2023). Establishing clear communication channels and responsibilities early on is the best practice for smooth operational flow in any multi-site study (Cummins et al., 2023). Utilizing project management tools and routinely revisiting timelines and resource needs would adaptively benefit future large-scale fieldwork (see also Cummins et al., 2023).

Adapting to Local Contexts

Sampling strategies in GUIDE are tailored to each country's linguistic, cultural, and geographic context, while accounting for feasible cross-country comparison (Babarović et al., 2025; Babarović et al., 2025). Pilot samples consider key population characteristics but need not be nationally representative (see Chap. 4 in this book). Local adaptations help improve participation and data quality while staying aligned with GUIDE protocols. Other projects conducting cross-cultural or multi-regional surveys should emphasize culturally sensitive survey design and data collection approaches (Babarović et al., 2025; Babarović et al., 2025). Piloting instruments with local samples and involving cultural experts enhances validity. Employing translation/back-translation and cognitive testing methods is widely recommended for ensuring questions are understood equivalently across contexts (Babarović et al., 2025).

Resource Management across Locations

In GUIDE, resource use—staff, mode of data collection, incentives—is planned according to country size and infrastructure (Babarović et al., 2025). National teams manage pilots and recruitment together with agencies (see also Chap. 5 in this book). Regular collaboration between all parties ensures efficiency and consistency across sites. Effective resource allocation according to local capabilities and constraints is vital in any decentralized or multi-site project (see also Briceno-Rosas et al., 2020). Leveraging centralized procurement or shared service models can optimize costs and quality (Briceno-Rosas et al., 2020). Establishing common quality standards while allowing flexibility in operational details supports scalability. Frequent coordination meetings and real-time progress tracking tools aid in managing diverse teams and sites.

Data Collection Methods

This section describes the range of data collection modes employed by large-scale longitudinal studies, highlighting their benefits, limitations, and situational uses (Dangubic & Voorpostel, 2017). Prominent data collection methods used in large longitudinal studies are discussed in detail including; Computer-Assisted Video Interviewing (CAVI); online survey tools; mobile technologies, examining both passive (automatic data collection) and active (user-engaged) methods; telephone interviews, exploring techniques for remote verbal data gathering; online interviews, covering video conferencing tools for face-to-face remote interactions; and in-person interviews, discussing strategies for direct, personal data collection. Table 3.2 contains brief descriptions of prominent data collection methods used in large longitudinal studies.

Box 3.1 Common Data Collection Methods

Computer-assisted personal interviewing (CAPI) is carried out through in-person interviews, where interviewers use electronic devices such as tablets or laptops to conduct surveys and record answers directly during the interaction.

Computer-Assisted Video Interviewing (CAVI) has the interviewer conduct the interview through video-call services (e.g., Teams, Zoom, Google Meets) while simultaneously logging the answers into software. These methods are also referred to in research literature as Video Mediated Interviews (VMI) (Rossetti et al., 2025).

Computer-assisted telephone interviewing (CATI) involves survey administration over the phone, where trained interviewers ask questions and enter responses directly into the research platform in use.

Online survey tools involve web-based surveys completed by respondents via computers or mobile devices through online platforms (SurveyMonkey, Google forms, Qualtrics, RedCap, Webropol), enabling automatic data collection without the involvement of an interviewer.

Personal Mobile technologies Passive mobile data collection involves the automatic mobile collection of data through sensors or apps running in the background on mobile devices, requiring minimal user input. Active user-engaged mobile data collection involves participants engaging directly with their devices, such as completing surveys or diary entries using mobile apps or web forms, often complementing CAVI methods.

Computer-Assisted Personal Interviewing

Computer-Assisted Personal Interviewing (CAPI) involves face-to-face interviews where interviewers use electronic devices (e.g., tablets and laptops) to administer surveys and record responses on-site. CAPI provides the richest data quality, particularly for complex surveys requiring explanations, probing, or use of visual aids. It allows inclusion of individuals without internet or phone access, reaching diverse populations. However, it has higher costs and logistical demands due to interviewer travel and longer administration time.

Computer-Assisted Video Interviewing

Computer-Assisted Video Interviewing (CAVI) involves the interviewer conducting the interview through video conferencing tools (e.g., Teams, Zoom, Google Meets) while simultaneously logging the answers into software. These methods are also referred to in research literature as Video Mediated Interviews (VMI; Rossetti et al., 2025). Video conferencing tool platforms allow real-time face-to-face interviews conducted remotely via video calls (Teams, Zoom, Google Forms), combining visual cues and interviewer interaction. Online interviews enable qualitative data collection through direct interaction, albeit remotely, offering a balance between reach, depth of insight, and cost effectiveness. The main advantages of CAVI are its broad geographic reach and reaching otherwise hard-to-reach groups, such as stay-at-home parents, migrant workers, and people in vulnerable living conditions. Other benefits include cost-efficiency due to automation and elimination of interviewer travel expenses, and the high level of privacy it offers respondents. CAVI is particularly effective for simple, straightforward surveys and enables rapid data collection.

Computer-Assisted Telephone Interviewing

Computer-Assisted Telephone Interviewing (CATI) systems involve trained interviewers who administer surveys over the phone with data entered directly into software. Telephone interviewing allows interviewers to clarify questions and probe further, offering more detailed data than web-based surveys but less than in-person methods. It has a broader reach than face-to-face interviews but excludes segments without phone access and can be limited by call scheduling and respondent availability.

Online Survey Tools

Online Survey Tools are web-based tools used to complete surveys by respondents via computers or mobile devices. These surveys are self-administered through online platforms (SurveyMonkey, Google Forms, Qualtrics, RedCap, and Webropol) that allow for automated data collection without the need for an interviewer present. However, because online survey tools lack an interviewer, they typically provide less opportunity for in-depth qualitative probing, which limits detailed insights compared to interviewer-led methods.

Personal Mobile Technologies

Data Collection with Personal Mobile Technologies involves the automatic mobile collection of data through sensors or apps running in the background on mobile devices, requiring minimal user input. Active User-Engaged mobile data collection involves participants engaging directly with their devices, such as completing surveys or diary entries using mobile apps or web forms, often complementing CAVI methods.

Examples of Data Collection in Practice from Large European Longitudinal Studies

In practice, CAPI has been widely used to enhance the efficiency, accuracy, and security of large-scale survey data collection. For example, in the Growing Up in Ireland study, interviewers administered questionnaires on laptops, reading questions aloud and directly entering responses, which minimized errors associated with manual data entry (Counihan et al., 2023). The interview software allowed for automated routing of questions, so that irrelevant items were skipped, and incorporated consistency and range checks to flag improbable responses. Participants were also supported with prompt cards to help navigate long or complex lists of response options. Once completed, interviews were encrypted, securely uploaded to a central server, and later converted into formats suitable for statistical analysis, ensuring both confidentiality and streamlined data processing (Counihan et al., 2023).

CAVI methods are increasingly being applied in practice to complement or substitute traditional face-to-face data collection. In the Italian Labor Force Survey experiment, CAVI-interviews (Video Mediated Interviews, referred to as VMI in the study) were conducted through secure platforms such as Microsoft Teams, allowing interviewers to connect with respondents in real time without requiring physical visits (Rossetti et al., 2025). This approach enabled researchers to reach individuals who were difficult to contact in person, such as those working full-time or living in remote areas, while also reducing costs and delays (Rossetti et al., 2025). Respondents were contacted initially in person to schedule and explain the video conference, followed by reminders sent via SMS with a secure meeting link. During interviews, both interviewer and respondent were encouraged to keep cameras on to replicate face-to-face interaction, though participation with video was optional. The study showed that VMIs could successfully collect objective data such as employment status and household information with accuracy comparable to CAPI (Rossetti et al., 2025).

Adapting Methodologies to a Child-Centered Context

Methodologies can be adapted to center on children's perspectives, ensuring their participation is meaningful and age-appropriate (e.g., participatory activities, tailored survey instruments). Such adaptations are essential for collecting valid data from children (Babarović et al., 2025). Child-centered methods prioritize children's own perspectives, recognizing that their views differ from those of adults and are essential for understanding wellbeing (see Chap. 1 in this book). Large studies like GUIDE will demonstrate that children's wellbeing can inform social policies by directly engaging 8-year-olds through harmonized surveys and CAPI and CAVI interviewing. While this approach captures children's voices across countries, it also faces challenges, including children's limited reading and communication skills, difficulties interpreting abstract survey items, and the need for validated instruments in multiple languages (Babarović et al., 2025). GUIDE follows the below best practices for child-centered fieldwork (Babarović et al., 2025; Foster et al., 2025; TENK, 2020):

Best Practices for Child-Centered Fieldwork

- **Build rapport and trust**: Begin with simple, friendly interactions; ensure interviewers are trained to communicate empathetically and at the child's level.

- **Adapt language and tools**: Use short, concrete questions, age-appropriate vocabulary, visual aids, and scales with pictorial options (e.g., smiley faces) to aid comprehension.
- **Ensure voluntary participation**: Emphasize that children can skip questions or stop at any time, reinforcing autonomy and ethical standards.
- **Use interviewer-administered methods**: For younger children, avoid self-completion formats; read questions aloud and confirm understanding.
- **Pilot test instruments**: Validate questionnaires with children of the target age group, across languages and cultures, before large-scale rollout.
- **Cultural and linguistic adaptation**: Employ child-friendly translations and ensure questions reflect culturally relevant experiences.
- **Create a safe environment**: Conduct interviews in familiar settings (schools, homes) and ensure privacy.
- **Monitor cognitive load**: Keep sessions short, include breaks, and limit the number of abstract or repetitive items.

Further Recommendations for Survey Development (Babarović et al., 2025)

- Invest in **cross-national instrument validation** for children to ensure comparability (see Chap. 9 in this book).
- Prioritize **developmentally appropriate design** over simply adapting adult-focused tools.
- Train interviewers not just technically but also in **child engagement strategies**.
- Combine **quantitative survey items with qualitative elements** (e.g., drawings or open-ended prompts) to capture richer perspectives.

Child-centered fieldwork practices enhance reliability, respect children's agency, make participation meaningful, and ensure data truly reflects children's experiences.

Training and Monitoring Field Researchers

To successfully implement a child-centered methodology, fieldworkers require specific training and monitoring. As the face of the project, their conduct directly shapes participant trust, comfort, and long-term retention (ALLEA, 2017). Training should go beyond procedural compliance (such as administering consent) and foster a deep, practical understanding of child-centered research (Crivello & Morrow, 2021). Cultural competence is also central (cf. Third et al., 2025), and fieldworker training should cover diverse cultural expectations; lessons from projects such as Born in Bradford (bilingual staff; Wright et al., 2013) and Roma inclusion projects (engaging gatekeepers; Condon et al., 2019) show that cultural sensitivity is a prerequisite for genuine inclusion.

GUIDE's training will be built on the COORDINATE project's model: centralized training resources complemented by country-specific modules co-designed with local partners.

Core Training Competencies

- **Rights-Based Foundations:** UNCRC principles, child agency, and protection.
- **Informed Consent/Assent:** Practical role-play for age-appropriate, layered approaches.
- **Cultural Competence:** Handling local norms around childhood, family, and authority.
- **Handling Distress:** Protocols for responding sensitively to child or parent discomfort.
- **Safeguarding:** Recognizing and reporting child protection concerns.
- **Data Protection:** Secure handling of sensitive data per GDPR.
- **Situated Ethics:** Awareness of power dynamics and handling field dilemmas.

In practice, GUIDE will rely on professional fieldwork agencies (e.g., Ipsos, Kantar). Since multiple contractors will be used, GUIDE should establish clear, non-negotiable standards. While agencies train their staff, GUIDE will supply the core content: detailed ethical guidance, scenario-based protocols, and minimum competency requirements. Oversight mechanisms, such as joint training sessions and quality audits, are essential to ensure alignment.

Ongoing monitoring is vital to handle dilemmas in the field. Key mechanisms include:

- **Supervisory Structures:** Regular debriefing sessions for fieldworkers.
- **Practice Audits:** Spot checks and participant feedback.
- **Transparent Reporting:** Clear channels for children and families to raise concerns.

Future Trends in Data Collection Techniques

Data collection is shifting toward greater digitalization (Facca et al., 2020), with increased use of online platforms and digital survey tools that streamline logistics, lower costs, and expand reach—though researchers remain attentive to data security, privacy, and digital exclusion issues. FAIR data principles (see Chap. 8 in this book) promote standardized data formats and interoperability across projects and countries (Jacobsen et al., 2020). Adaptive sampling, real-time digital dashboards, AI-powered survey instruments, and integration with administrative datasets are emerging as best practices, supporting better coverage of diverse and hard-to-reach groups (see also Whitmeyer et al., 2019).

Expanding digitalization needs to be increasingly accounted for in child-centered research. Future directions in research on digitalization and child wellbeing emphasize a nuanced understanding of both positive and negative impacts of technology on children's lives (Facca et al., 2020; Internet Matters, 2025). Recent findings highlight growing polarization: while many children benefit socially from digital connectivity, vulnerable groups face heightened risks and negative experiences online, such as increased exposure to upsetting content and safety concerns (Internet Matters, 2025). Key future research priorities concerning digitalization include topics such as the following (Facca et al., 2020; Internet Matters, 2025):

- **Addressing Inequalities** in digital access and experiences, focusing on vulnerable or marginalized children.
- **Developing Nuanced Measures** to capture complex digital constructs, beyond screen time alone, including social connectedness, emotional response, and agency in digital use.
- **Fostering Interdisciplinary Approaches** to integrating psychology, education, human-computer interaction, and policy to design supportive digital environments tailored to developmental needs.
- **Exploring Emerging Digital Formats** such as adaptive learning technologies (Molenaar, 2021) and digital mental health interventions, assessing impacts on behavior, cognition, and socioemotional development.
- **Co-Designing Technologies with Children** to ensure that tools promote autonomy, creativity, and safety, empowering children as active digital citizens rather than passive consumers.
- **Enhancing Parental and Educator Digital Literacy and Mediation**, supporting informed guidance and boundary-setting without undermining children's agency or privacy.
- **Investigating Periodical Shifts** in digital engagement patterns and long-term consequences for wellbeing, learning, and social development.

Digital transformation includes use of secure cloud storage, electronic communication, and advanced data management, promoting accessibility and collaborative analysis. Systematic training and training of national and local teams are prioritized, ensuring methodological consistency and responsiveness to new digital research environments. New modes such as audio-enhanced surveys, app-based diary studies, and video-enabled interviews expand methodological options while accommodating respondents' preferences and constraints (Alcaire et al., 2024; Brigidi & Leyva-Moral, 2025). In summary, future research on digital child wellbeing will be increasingly participatory, interdisciplinary, and equity-oriented, with a strong focus on integrating children's perspectives in the development of safe, enriching digital experiences and evidence-based policies that promote holistic wellbeing in an evolving digital landscape.

Emerging Practices on Digital Child-Centered Research

Digital child-centered research methods prioritize children's voices, agencies, and perspectives within digital contexts, recognizing children as active participants shaped by and shaping their digital environments. These methods include participatory and observational techniques adapted to technological affordances, such as digital walk-throughs where children share their screen activity or react to digital stimuli in real time, which increases ecological validity and captures authentic digital experiences. Ethical challenges include managing privacy, unexpected disclosures, consent complexities, and risks of exposure to harmful content, which require clear protocols for confidentiality, mandatory reporting, and child safety (see Chap. 2 in this book; Facca et al., 2020; Internet Matters, 2025; Kucirkova et al., 2024; Livingstone & Locatelli, 2012). Based on the above-mentioned literature, the following recommendations for best practices can be established:

Recommendations and Best Practices for Digital Child-Centered Fieldwork

- **Ensure Privacy and Data Protection:** Use secure platforms and encrypted data storage; obtain informed consent that clearly explains digital risks and confidentiality limits.
- **Build Rapport Digitally:** Train interviewers to engage children warmly via video or audio, using child-friendly digital interfaces that reduce barriers to communication.
- **Adapt Instruments Digitally:** Employ multimedia tools such as animated visuals, interactive scales (e.g., smiley faces), and audio prompts to support comprehension.
- **Use Hybrid Methods:** Combine surveys, diaries, observations, and qualitative inputs (e.g., video diaries) to capture a richer picture of children's experiences with technology.
- **Address Accessibility:** Consider children's digital literacy levels, device access, and socio-economic and linguistic diversity when designing studies.
- **Plan for Digital Ethics:** Anticipate and prepare for disclosures of harm or illegal content by children, balancing child privacy with safeguarding responsibilities.
- **Engage Children as Co-Researchers:** Involve children in the design and interpretation phases, empowering participation and ensuring methods align with lived realities.
- **Pilot and Validate:** Test digital methods and translations thoroughly for diverse child populations to ensure reliability and cross-cultural relevance.
- **Promote Inclusiveness:** Recruit diverse samples, including those with special educational needs or limited digital access, to avoid bias and increase equity.

By integrating these practices, digital child-centered research can produce ethically sound, developmentally appropriate, and methodologically rigorous data that reflect children's genuine experiences in a rapidly changing digital world.

Summary of Key Insights and Lessons Learned for the First Wave of GUIDE

As part of the preparatory phase of GUIDE, the development of the GUIDE survey methodology is a core objective. This includes finalizing the design of GUIDE sampling and recruitment strategies, developing and refining the questionnaires, and establishing detailed fieldwork procedures. Rigorous fieldwork planning, ethical oversight, continuous monitoring, and quality control are foundational to support Wave 1 of GUIDE fieldwork. The Central Hub plans to coordinate fieldwork activities, providing standardized protocols, training, and quality control procedures. It will work closely with national teams, who will be responsible for implementing the fieldwork locally in collaboration with survey agencies appointed.

Mixed-mode data collection is vital for inclusivity and flexibility, ensuring coverage of populations with varied digital and geographical access, including Computer-Assisted Video Interviewing for web-based interviews, enabling broad reach and cost-effectiveness; and Computer-Assisted Personal Interviewing for in-person interviews, suitable for complex questionnaires and reaching participants without reliable internet access.

GUIDE plans for fieldwork are centrally coordinated through the Central Hub, managing protocols and quality control and national teams executing fieldwork. This collaboration enables standardized, high-quality mixed-mode data collection, ensuring the first Waves of GUIDE are methodologically robust, culturally sensitive, and inclusive of diverse populations across Europe.

References

Alcaire, R., Flores, A. M. M., & Antunes, E. (2024). Beyond words: Tapping the potential of digital diaries while exploring young adults' experiences on apps. *Societies, 14*(3), Article 40. https://doi.org/10.3390/soc14030040

ALLEA. (2017). *The European Code of Conduct for Research Integrity*. https://allea.org/code-of-conduct/

Babarović, T., Krpanec, E., Blažev, M., & Černja Rajter, I. (2025). Developing an international, longitudinal questionnaire to study child wellbeing. In Editor(s) Initial(s). Last Name(s) (Ed[s].), *Title of the book* (pp. xx–xx). Publisher.

Babarović, T., Krpanec, E., Blažev, M., Dević, I., Downey, S., Huttunen, I. E., Panico, L., Perron, Z., Santos, A., Taylor, L. K., Upadyaya, K., Symonds, J., & Pollock, G. (2025). Children's understanding of Well-being related questions: Results of cognitive interviews in four European countries. *International Journal of Social Research Methodology, 28*(2), 163–178. https://doi.org/10.1080/13645579.2024.2312621

Babarović, T., Krpanec, E., Černja Rajter, I., Surdey, J., & Sloan, S. (2025). *Fieldwork manual & training*. European Union.

Biswas, K., Carty, C., Horney, R., Nasrin, D., Farag, T. H., Kotloff, K. L., & Levine, M. M. (2012). Data management and other logistical challenges for the GEMS: The data coordinating center perspective. *Clinical Infectious Diseases, 55*(Suppl. 4), S254–S261. https://doi.org/10.1093/cid/cis755

Briceno-Rosas, R., Butt, S., & Kappelhof, J. (2020). Improving central monitoring of fieldwork in cross-national surveys: The case of the fieldwork management system in the European Social Survey. *Survey Methods: Insights from the Field*. https://surveyinsights.org/?p=11866

Brigidi, S., & Leyva-Moral, J. M. (2025). Capturing lived experiences remotely: Exploring the potential of audio diaries as an innovative qualitative data collection method in crisis contexts. *Kontakt, 27*(2), 117–122. https://doi.org/10.32725/kont.2025.005

Broekstra, R., Aris-Meijer, J., Maeckelberghe, E., Stolk, R., & Otten, S. (2020). Trust in centralized large-scale data repository: A qualitative analysis. *Journal of Empirical Research on Human Research Ethics, 15*(4), 365–378. https://doi.org/10.1177/1556264619888365

Condon, L., Bedford, H., Ireland, L., Kerr, S., Mytton, J., Richardson, Z., & Jackson, C. (2019). Engaging gypsy, Roma, and Traveller communities in research: Maximizing opportunities and overcoming challenges. *Qualitative Health Research, 29*(9), 1324–1333. https://doi.org/10.1177/1049732318813558

Counihan, D., O'Shea, M. T., Guigui, D., Sloan, S., Chzen, Y., Taylor, L. K., & Symonds, J. E. (2023). Scoping review to inform the development of a potential new birth cohort for growing up in Ireland. Department of Children, Equality, Disability, Integration and Youth. https://www.growingup.gov.ie/pubs/230525-GUI-Scoping-Review.pdf

Crivello, G., & Morrow, V. (2021). *Ethics learning from Young Lives: 20 years on*. Young Lives. https://www.younglives.org.uk/publications/ethics-learning-young-lives-20-years

Cummins, M. R., Burr, J., Young, L., Yeatts, S. D., Ecklund, D. J., Bunnell, B. E., Dwyer, J. P., & VanBuren, J. M. (2023). Decentralized research technology use in multicenter clinical research studies based at U.S. academic research centers. *Journal of Clinical and Translational Science*, 7(1), e250. doi:https://doi.org/10.1017/cts.2023.678.

Dangubic, M., & Voorpostel, M. (2017). *Computer-assisted web interviewing (CAWI) in the Swiss household panel: Demographics, participation and data quality* (Swiss household panel working paper 1_17).

Facca, D., Smith, M. J., Shelley, J., Lizotte, D., & Donelle, L. (2020). Exploring the ethical issues in research using digital data collection strategies with minors: A scoping review. *PLoS One, 15*(8), e0237875. https://doi.org/10.1371/journal.pone.0237875

Foster, M., Whitehead, L. L., O'Sullivan, T. A., Hill, J., & Mörelius, E. (2025). A child-centred research checklist to improve the design and reporting of paediatric research studies: A descriptive mixed methods study. *International Journal of Nursing Studies, 162*, 104958. https://doi.org/10.1016/j.ijnurstu.2024.104958

Hanke, M., Pestilli, F., Wagner, A. S., Markiewicz, C. J., Poline, J. B., & Halchenko, Y. O. (2021). In defense of decentralized research data management. *e-Neuroforum, 27*(1), 17–25. https://doi.org/10.1515/nf-2020-0037

Internet Matters. (2025). *Children's wellbeing in a digital world 2025: Year 4 annual index report*. https://www.internetmatters.org/hub/research/childrens-wellbeing-in-a-digital-world-index-report-2025/

Islam, S., & Apu, K. U. (2024). Decentralized vs. centralized database solutions in blockchain: Advantages, challenges, and use cases. *Global Mainstream Journal of Innovation, Engineering & Emerging Technology, 3*(4), 58–68. https://doi.org/10.62304/jieet.v3i04.195

Jacobsen, A., de Miranda Azevedo, R., Juty, N., Batista, D., Coles, S., Cornet, R., Courtot, M., Crosas, M., Dumontier, M., Evelo, C. T., Goble, C., Guizzardi, G., Hansen, K. K., Hasnain, A., Hettne, K., Heringa, J., Hooft, R. W. W., Imming, M., Jeffery, K. G., et al. (2020). FAIR principles: Interpretations and implementation considerations. *Data Intelligence, 2*(1–2), 10–29. https://doi.org/10.1162/dint_r_00024

Khalilov, E. (2023). *To understand the complexities of centralized and decentralized approaches in managing organizational change and innovation*. University of Lodz. https://https://doi.org/10.13140/RG.2.2.17776.02565

Kucirkova, N., Livingstone, S., & Radesky, J. (2024). Advancing the understanding of children's digital engagement: Responsive methodologies and ethical considerations in psychological research. *Frontiers in Psychology, 15*, 1285302. https://doi.org/10.3389/fpsyg.2024.1285302

Leung, L. (2015). Validity, reliability, and generalizability in qualitative research. *Journal of Family Medicine and Primary Care, 4*(3), 324–327. https://doi.org/10.4103/2249-4863.161306

Livingstone, S., & Locatelli, E. (2012). Ethical dilemmas in qualitative research with youth on/offline. *International Journal of Learning and Media, 4*(2), 67–75. https://doi.org/10.1162/IJLM_a_00096

Mang, J., Küchenhoff, H., & Meinck, S. (2024). Evaluating German PISA stratification designs: A simulation study. *Large-Scale Assessments in Education, 12*, 15. https://doi.org/10.1186/s40536-024-00203-0

Molenaar, I. (2021). Personalization of learning: Towards hybrid human-AI learning technologies. *Blockchain, and Robots*, 57–77.

Rossetti, F., Bontempi, K., & Pietropaoli, S. (2025). A comparison between video mediated interview (VMI) and CAPI in labour force survey. *Metron, 83*, 75–91. https://doi.org/10.1007/s40300-024-00282-7

TENK (Finnish National Board on Research Integrity). (2020). *Guidelines for ethical review in human sciences*. https://tenk.fi/en/advice-and-materials/guidelines-ethical-review-human-sciences

Third, A., Baú, V., Tasker, S., & Welland, L. (2025). *Involving children in research and data collection: A gap analysis*. Save the Children International. https://resourcecentre.savethechildren.net/pdf/FINAL_Gap-Analysis-research-brief_25.03.2025.pdf

Upadyaya, K., Huttunen, I., Surdey, J., & Sloan, S. (2025). *Fieldwork costings*. European Union.

Whitmeyer, S. J., Pyle, E. J., Pavlis, T. L., Swanger, W., & Roberts, L. (2019). Modern approaches to field data collection and mapping: Digital methods, crowdsourcing, and the future of statistical analyses. *Journal of Structural Geology, 125*, 29–40. https://doi.org/10.1016/j.jsg.2018.06.023

Wright, J., Small, N., Raynor, P., Tuffnell, D., Bhopal, R., Cameron, N., Fairley, L., Lawlor, D. A., Parslow, R., Petherick, E. S., Pickett, K. E., Waiblinger, D., West, J., & Born in Bradford Scientific Collaborators Group. (2013). Cohort profile: The born in Bradford multi-ethnic family cohort study. International Journal of Epidemiology, 42(4), 978–991. doi:https://doi.org/10.1093/ije/dys112.

Katja Upadyaya (Ph.D.) is a research director at the University of Helsinki's Faculty of Educational Sciences. Her research focuses on academic and occupational wellbeing, motivation, teacher-student and parent-child interactions, as well as children's wellbeing, socio-emotional skills, and parental burnout, resilience, and future preparedness. She also specializes in research methodology.

Arttu Brax (MAEd) is a technical assistant with a background in educational psychology and teacher training. He is currently working in the University of Helsinki branch of EDUCA, the educational sciences flagship project of the Research Council of Finland. His work examines the school environment's effect on student wellbeing and the use of ICT and AI in education.

Stephanie Cahill (Ph.D.) is a research associate at Manchester Metropolitan University, specializing in child and adolescent wellbeing, life course perspectives, and resilience. Her current research explores children's digital wellbeing, the impact of climate change on mental health, and ethical considerations in research involving children and young people.

Chapter 4
Selecting and Retaining Representative Longitudinal Infant and Child Cohort Samples

Gaspar Massiot and Shuang Su

Examining the developmental trajectory of children's wellbeing in a cross-national, longitudinal study like GUIDE requires robust sampling methodologies that are closely coordinated to ensure comparability. Such an ambitious approach presents significant challenges in ensuring that samples are accurately selected across different countries. This chapter outlines the proposed cohort design for GUIDE, structured around a five-step framework rooted in established methodological principles. The discussion proceeds through each step of the design, ranging from defining the target population to managing longitudinal retention. For each step, the discussion integrates comparative insights from leading European longitudinal studies (e.g., ESS, SHARE, NEPS). These case-based lessons are then directly applied to inform the GUIDE approach. The final section summarizes the design's strengths alongside future directions and challenges.

A Five-Step Framework for Longitudinal, Cross-National Research

GUIDE's framework is informed by established best practices, including the benchmark in cross-national research (Hubbard et al., 2016), and "lessons learned" from other leading European studies (see Table 4.1). To select an optimal sample in each participating country that is representative of the target population and of sufficient

G. Massiot (✉)
Institut National d'Etudes Démographiques (INED), Aubervilliers, France
e-mail: Gaspar.massiot@ined.fr

S. Su
School of Education, University College Dublin, Dublin, Ireland

L. K. Taylor et al. (eds.), *Growing Up in Digital Europe*, Springer Series on Child and Family Studies, https://doi.org/10.1007/978-3-032-30592-3_4

quality for robust scientific inference, the following sections detail each of the five steps:

1. Define the *target population* for the study across all countries and the *survey population* within each participating country (Hubbard et al., 2016, para. 1).
2. Identify and evaluate potential *sampling frames*. Select or create the sampling frame that best covers the target population for each participating country (Hubbard et al., 2016, para. 1).
3. Choose a *selection procedure* that will randomly select units from the sampling frame and ensure that important subgroups in the population will be represented (Hubbard et al., 2016, para. 1).
4. Determine the *sample size* necessary to meet the desired level of precision for the statistics of interest at population or subgroup levels based on the sample selection procedures (Hubbard et al., 2016, para. 1).
5. Implement longitudinal *retention and attrition management* to maintain the effective sample size over time (cf. Fokkema et al., 2016; Gauthier et al., 2018).

For each step, we first discuss the relevant best practices derived from other European studies and then outline the specific GUIDE approach. We conclude by reviewing the links to quality control in fieldwork (see Chap. 3 in this book) and documentation to support open science (see Chap. 8 in this book).

Step 1: Target and Survey Population

Best Practices and Methodological Considerations

A distinction must be made between the *target population* (i.e., the finite population we ideally want to investigate; Groves et al., 2011) and the *survey population* (i.e., the group from which we can realistically collect data; Hubbard et al., 2016). The target population specifies the units and time frame, such as all children of a given age residing in the country at the time of the study (Groves et al., 2011). The survey population is a restricted set of these units, often limited by cost, access, or security constraints. This distinction can be viewed as "who we want to include in our survey" versus "who we can include in our survey" (Hubbard et al., 2016, Guidelines section, para. 5).

For cross-national surveys, a detailed, concise definition of the target population is essential to ensure that each participating country collects data from the same population, which underpins harmonization and comparability (see Chap. 9 in this book; Hubbard et al., 2016; Jabkowski & Kołczyńska, 2020; T. W. Smith, 2018). For example, exclusion criteria around the target population might include people who are homeless, those living in institutions such as hospitals or prisons, or those who cannot speak the official national language(s) (Bergmann et al., 2017; De Luca et al., 2015).

Table 4.1 Summary of eight European Cross-National (ESS, SHARE, EU-SILC, GGS) or longitudinal studies (MoBa, ELFE, NEPS, GUI)

Study name and citation	Target population	Sampling frame	Sample selection procedure	Target sample size	Retention and attrition management
The European Social Survey (ESS; Häder et al., 2003; Lynn et al., 2007)	All people aged 15 and over resident within private households, regardless of nationality, citizenship, language, or legal status.	Individual/household registers or address lists.	Two-stage random sampling (stage 1: Municipalities; stage 2: Households).	Effective size 1500 (800 for populations under two million); minimum net size 2000; target response rate 70%.	Advance letters; toll-free contact numbers; interviewer training on response maximization techniques.
The Survey of Health, Ageing and Retirement in Europe (SHARE; Bergmann et al., 2017; Bergmann & Scherpenzeel, 2016)	People aged 50 years or older regularly domiciled in the respective country.	Official population registers covering the target population.	Multi-stage stratified probability sampling.	Net sample size determined by available budget; countries aim to maximize net size (no universal minimum requirement).	Continuous fieldwork monitoring, including assessment of interviewer performance and panel member response behavior.
The European Union Statistics on Income and Living Conditions (EU-SILC; Eurostat, 2023)	All people residing in private households within the national territory (longitudinally tracked across subsequent waves).	National population registers or address/census lists.	Probability sampling (varies by country: Simple random, stratified, or multi-stage sampling).	Over 200,000 households annually (covering >500,000 individuals).	Rotational panel design; tracing rules; longitudinal weighting.
The Generation and Gender Survey (GGS; Fokkema et al., 2016; Gauthier et al., 2018)	Non-institutionalized residents aged 18–79 (at wave 1).	Population registers (individuals) or area/dwelling frames.	Probability sampling (1–3 stages); stratified, simple random, probability proportional to size, or random route.	Minimum 10,000 at wave 1 (aiming for 8000 by wave 3); average response rate 56%.	Incentives; regular contact (including annual short questionnaires); interviewer continuity; specialized training.

(continued)

Table 4.1 (continued)

Study name and citation	Target population	Sampling frame	Sample selection procedure	Target sample size	Retention and attrition management
The Norwegian Mother and Child Cohort Study (MoBa; Magnus et al., 2006, 2016; MoBa, 2025)	All women who give birth in Norway (recruited 1999–2008).	Routine ultrasound examination lists (the pregnancy is the unit of observation).	Inclusion of all maternity units with more than 100 annual births (52 units).	95,369 pregnant women.	Passive tracking via national registry; feedback loop (newsletters); multi-mode reminders
The French Longitudinal Study of Children (ELFE; Charles et al., 2020; Elfe, 2025; Pirus et al., 2010)	All mothers giving birth in metropolitan France (mainland and Corsica).	Newborns in 349 randomly sampled maternity units.	Stratified sampling (allocation proportional to maternity unit size).	Final sample 18,329 infants.	Dedicated website; small birthday gifts; close monitoring of nonresponse reasons.
The German National Educational Panel Study (NEPS; Anger et al., 2019; Schaeper, 2013; Zinn et al., 2020)	Six starting cohorts (SC1–SC6): Newborns; kindergarten children; fifth graders; ninth graders; first-year university students; adults (born 1944–1986).	Institutional lists (schools/universities) or population registers (newborns/adults).	Multi-stage stratified cluster sampling (institutions); direct stratified probability sampling (individuals).	Total > 60,000 participants. Individual cohorts range from ~3500 (newborns) to ~18,000 (first-year university students).	Active individual tracing; incentives; flexible interview modes; adaptive survey intervals; regular newsletters.
Growing Up in Ireland (the Cohort '08 of GUI; Quail et al., 2011)	41,185 infants registered on the Child Benefit Register as having been born between first December 2007 and 30th June 2008.	The child benefit register and vital statistics in Ireland.	Random sampling.	11,134 nine-month-old children.	Participant tracing; active contact; interviewer consistency; flexible data collection; statistical weighting.

GUIDE's Approach

GUIDE is an accelerated cohort study with two distinct target populations: the Child Cohort (residents aged 8 years) and the Infant Cohort (residents aged 6 to 9 months). The primary inclusion criteria are age and residency. This includes children whose families are temporarily away from the country for less than 6 months, for reasons such as a holiday. Furthermore, the Child Cohort's target population is not restricted to children currently attending mainstream school. To ensure feasibility, the design also applies specific exclusion criteria: (1) residents absent for 6 months or more; (2) temporary visitors/tourists; (3) children living in institutions; and (4) households where severe language barriers prevent informed consent. Finally, while children are the target population in both cohorts, for the Infant Cohort, only one legal representative is interviewed; each national team should ensure this person is best-suited to answer questions about the infant's health and development and document which parent or legal representative is interviewed (Blöss, 2009).

Step 2: Sampling Frame

Best Practices and Methodological Considerations

The *sampling frame* serves as the operational resource used to identify and contact the target population (Heeringa & O'muircheartaigh, 2010; Hubbard et al., 2016). Sampling frames can either be pre-existing (e.g., population register; Scherpenzeel et al., 2017) or be created via area probability sampling methods when no pre-existing list is available (e.g., sampling based on geographic information systems; Eckman et al., 2018). The primary quality criterion of a sampling frame is coverage—the degree of correspondence between the frame and the target population (Groves et al., 2011). Coverage errors manifest as either *under-coverage* (the exclusion of eligible units) or *over-coverage* (the inclusion of ineligible units) (Groves et al., 2011). Methodological best practice dictates that several potential frames are assessed for quality, suitability, and coverage during the planning stage. Once a frame is selected, it must be rigorously evaluated to mitigate structural defects, particularly clustering (where a single frame entry maps to multiple population units) and duplication (where a single population unit maps to multiple frame entries). Furthermore, the frame must be screened to identify and remove ineligible units (Groves et al., 2011). In sum, the importance of maximizing coverage should be emphasized, and frames should be updated in the timeliest manner possible.

In cross-national research, a common sampling frame rarely exists (Carfagna & Carfagna, 2015). This means countries could use the best available pre-existing lists, such as official population registries, health registries, or lists of schools (Scherpenzeel et al., 2017). The challenge is that not all countries have a comprehensive national register, which complicates harmonization (Scherpenzeel et al., 2017).

Sampling infants and children also present specific challenges. For infant cohorts, strategies have included recruiting pregnant women (Magnus et al., 2006; MoBa, 2025), sampling from maternity hospitals (Elfe, 2025; Pirus et al., 2010), or using municipality birth registers (Schaeper, 2013; Zinn et al., 2020) and national benefit registers (Quail et al., 2011). For older child cohorts, such as those in NEPS (Schaeper, 2013; Zinn et al., 2020) and GUI (Quail et al., 2011), school lists are a common frame, though this approach risks excluding unschooled children.

GUIDE's Approach

For GUIDE, sampling frames should provide a nonzero probability of selection for every eligible unit of the target population. As such, *list frames* (such as population registers) have an advantage over *area frames* (such as counties or city blocks). Moreover, a list frame should include key auxiliary variables: age, sex, and place of residence, along with tracing information such as the names of the child and legal guardian, phone numbers, and addresses (see Chapters 2 and 8 in this book), and ideally variables for nonresponse analysis (e.g., income, household size).

National teams should be aware that access to all potential sampling frames may need to be negotiated, allocating sufficient time and resources in early planning stages. For the Child Cohort, school rolls may be used, but they should be complemented with another appropriate frame to avoid the under-coverage of unschooled children. For the Infant Cohort, population registers, birth registers, and health-service registers are the most likely to provide good coverage; yet access to these lists is a known challenge in many countries. For this cohort, if access to these registers is not possible, national teams might consider developing collaborations with medical professionals in newborn or prenatal care (Magnus et al., 2006; Pirus et al., 2010).

Step 3: Sample Selection Procedures

Best Practices and Methodological Considerations

Once a sampling frame is established, a *selection procedure* is required. This procedure should rely on *probability sampling* defined as a method where every unit (e.g., person, household) in the target population has a known, nonzero probability of selection (Pace, 2021). This approach is the "gold standard" for quantitative research (Kalton, 2023), allowing for valid statistical inference, the calculation of sampling errors, and the minimization of selection bias (Heeringa & O'muircheartaigh, 2010).

In practice, the choice of a specific probability sampling method involves a trade-off between precision and logistical efficiency. *Stratified sampling* is often employed to ensure good representation of specific subgroups (strata) (Jensen, 1991; Neyman,

1992), while *cluster sampling* is used to reduce costs for face-to-face interviews by sampling geographically constrained groups (Iqbal Jeelani et al., 2018). Although clustering improves fieldwork efficiency, it is less statistically precise and requires a larger sample size (Iqbal Jeelani et al., 2018).

The reviewed cross-national surveys show that selection procedures are not standardized across countries (see Table 4.1), as each adapted to the available national sampling frames (Scherpenzeel et al., 2017). Although all four cross-national studies (i.e., ESS, SHARE, EU-SILC, GGS) used probability sampling, methods ranged from direct Simple Random Sampling (SRS) or Systematic Random Sampling (SystRS) in countries with high-quality population registers to complex multi-stage, stratified, and clustered designs in other countries (Eurostat, 2023; Fokkema et al., 2016).

The reviewed birth and child cohorts also show diverse approaches. MoBa and ELFE used a form of complete enumeration within selected units, which means all women at a registry or all women in selected maternity wards will be included (Elfe, 2025; Magnus et al., 2006; MoBa, 2025; Pirus et al., 2010). The Cohort '08 of GUI, by contrast, used a true random selection procedure (stratified systematic sampling) from the national register, a methodology that is more suitable for a cross-national survey should a register be available (Quail et al., 2011).

GUIDE's Approach

GUIDE's sample should be selected by probability sampling methods (i.e., not quota sampling). Each participating country should consult with sampling experts to develop an optimal design that is appropriate for its national context, frame, and budget. For example, two likely options are multi-stage sampling and stratification. First, *multi-stage cluster designs* may be used to decrease fieldwork costs, particularly if the sampling frame is organized in clusters such as school lists (Groves et al., 2011; Hubbard et al., 2016). However, these cost savings are greatest for face-to-face interviewing and tend to decrease overtime in longitudinal surveys as the sample "de-clusters" when people move (Lynn, 2009). Given GUIDE's mixed-mode and longitudinal nature, potential cost savings from clustering may be limited and should be balanced against the loss in statistical precision (Hubbard et al., 2016). If multi-stage sampling is chosen, larger geographical areas should be preferred as primary sampling units, and a larger number of sampled units (e.g., schools) is preferred to a smaller number (Lynn, 2009). Second, proportionate *stratification* is highly beneficial and preferred over *simple random sampling* (i.e., every unit and combinations of units have the same probability of being selected when sampling), as it can improve the precision of sample estimates (Survey Research Center, 2010). Variables used for stratification (e.g., sex, age, and region) should be chosen based on their availability in the sampling frame and their association with the survey's key variables (see Chap. 5 in this book). The combined stratified multi-stage cluster designs could ensure adequate representation and facilitate more robust regional or subgroup estimates (Lynn, 2009; Survey Research Center, 2010).

Step 4: Determining Sample Size and Statistical Power

Best Practices and Methodological Considerations

Determining the target sample size is fundamental to ensuring the statistical precision of study estimates. The central metric in this process is the *effective sample size*—the number of participants required to achieve a specific level of precision if the study were using simple random sampling. To ensure cross-national comparability, for example, ESS mandates a uniform minimum effective sample size of 1500 for all participating nations (reduced to 800 for populations under two million) (Häder et al., 2003; Lynn et al., 2007). However, to achieve this target, the actual number of required interviews varies by country. This variance is dictated by the *design effect*, a metric that quantifies the loss of precision caused by complex sampling features such as clustering. By adjusting the sample size based on the national design effect, studies ensure consistent statistical power across all countries, regardless of their specific selection procedures (Häder et al., 2003; Lynn et al., 2007; Simard & Franklin, 2005).

For longitudinal studies, the most crucial factor is planning for attrition. The initial sample size at Wave 1 should be large enough to guarantee that even after years or decades of participant drop-out, the remaining sample is still statistically powerful enough for analysis (P. Smith et al., 2009). Therefore, the final *gross sample size* should account for the desired precision, the expected design effect, and the projected rates of nonresponse and attrition (Couper & Ofstedal, 2009).

GUIDE's Approach

To ensure that the later data collection waves of the study retain sufficient respondents for potential statistical analysis (see Chap. 9 in this book) based on reviewing related studies including ESS, larger countries might aim for a minimum effective sample size of 10,000 for the Infant Cohort and 8000 for the Child Cohort, and smaller countries (i.e., populations under ten million) might aim for 5000 for the Infant Cohort and 4000 for the Child Cohort.

Each country should calculate its own gross sample size by factoring in its specific sampling frame and sample design to reach the proposed effective sample size. This calculation requires estimating the design effect, the sample eligibility rate, and the expected Wave 1 response rate. Due to uncertainties over response rates, we recommend that a *reserve sample* be constructed in advance of fieldwork (Groves & Heeringa, 2006). The size of this reserve should be based on an estimate of the lowest response rate likely to be achieved with the main sample. For multiple reasons, countries may also want or need to over-sample targeted sub-populations due to particular policy interest or expected nonresponse (P. Smith et al., 2009). In this case, sampling weights will have to be used during analysis to ensure unbiased estimates of the total population (Valliant et al., 2013). Each country is strongly advised to consult with sampling experts to develop the optimal plan (Häder et al., 2003; Lynn et al., 2007).

Step 5: Longitudinal Retention and Attrition Management

Best Practices and Methodological Considerations

Once a sample is recruited, longitudinal retention becomes the most critical challenge (Lynn, 2020). Great care must be taken to control *attrition* (i.e., the loss of participants between waves) as it can reduce statistical power and jeopardize the integrity of the sample if certain groups drop out more than others (Zinn et al., 2020). Experience from other panels, such as the French GGS, shows that attrition is often highest between the first and second waves (Gauthier et al., 2018). Similarly, the NEPS SC1 (infant cohort) experienced a significant dropout between its first two waves (Schaeper, 2013; Zinn et al., 2020). This highlights the need for a robust retention strategy from the initiation of the survey.

Best practices for retention are multi-faceted: tracing, engagement, and monitoring. Tracing procedures are essential for locating participants who may move in different ways, such as collecting the contact information of another person unlikely to move (Schaeper, 2013; Zinn et al., 2020). Complementing this, engagement strategies aim to keep participants involved, such as sending regular survey newsletters, birthday cards, or asking participants to notify the survey agency of an address change (Quail et al., 2011; Schaeper, 2013; Zinn et al., 2020). Furthermore, many large-scale surveys also use monetary or non-financial incentives to encourage continued participation (Elfe, 2025; Fokkema et al., 2016; Gauthier et al., 2018; Pirus et al., 2010). Finally, rigorous fieldwork administration, including standardized interviewer training (Bergmann et al., 2017; Bergmann & Scherpenzeel, 2016; Häder et al., 2003; Lynn et al., 2007) and real-time monitoring of nonresponse patterns (Elfe, 2025; Magnus et al., 2006; MoBa, 2025; Pirus et al., 2010), is critical for identifying attrition risks early and ensuring the sustained viability of the survey.

GUIDE's Approach

GUIDE will strive to maintain the effective sample size over time through a multi-faceted tracing and retention strategy. For example, national teams should collect stable contact information (e.g., of a secondary contact person) at Wave 1. Furthermore, teams will maintain engagement with participants between waves through regular updates on survey findings, such as branded study newsletters. The use of modest, age-appropriate monetary or non-financial incentives to thank participants and maintain cooperation across waves is also recommended. Operationally, GUIDE will prioritize high-quality interviewer training and active fieldwork monitoring (see Chap. 3 in this book). Nonresponse at each wave will be closely monitored to better understand the reasons for attrition and develop responsive strategies (Mazen et al., 2019; Taylor et al., 2020).

Summary of Findings and Implications for GUIDE

This chapter suggests the need to critically balance cross-national comparability (see Chap. 9 in this book) with the practical realities of different national contexts. The five-step framework provides guidelines that empower each national team, in consultation with sampling experts and the central team, to develop an optimal design for their specific context to select and maintain high-quality, representative samples for comparative longitudinal analysis.

This framework is complemented by other chapters in this volume. First, from a sampling perspective, the primary goal of high-quality fieldwork is to achieve a high response rate while maintaining the integrity of the probability sample. Fieldwork *quality control* is essential for ensuring that the selected sample is successfully recruited and that the data is of the highest quality (see Chap. 3 in this book). This involves implementing *reproducibility standards*, such as creating a unique sample identification code for each unit and tracking key variables and outcomes (e.g., response status) throughout the entire sample lifecycle (Kreuter, 2013). Achieving a high initial response rate is a major challenge. For example, in Wave 1 of the GGS, the average response rate was 56%, with some countries experiencing much lower rates due to difficulties in contacting individuals and securing cooperation (Fokkema et al., 2016; Gauthier et al., 2018). To manage this, many studies use recruitment incentives (e.g., cash, vouchers, and lottery tickets) to stimulate initial participation (Fokkema et al., 2016; Gauthier et al., 2018). Other studies have used *Responsive Survey Designs* (RSDs). RSDs use data collected during fieldwork, such as response rates by region or nonresponse patterns, to guide mid-survey decisions (Groves & Heeringa, 2006; Tourangeau et al., 2017). Exploring such innovations might be particularly useful for GUIDE's Infant Cohort, which faces a narrow recruitment window.

Second, to promote Open Science (see Chap. 8 in this book), each country should *document* its sample design choices in a standardized report, including a description of the sampling frame used, including its limitations and any auxiliary variables; a definition of the survey population, noting the percentage of under-coverage and all exclusions; the Wave 1 sample size, with a description of its computation and the assumed nonresponse and attrition rates; a list of all stratification variables; the sample allocation across strata; and a detailed description of the final sample design and its specific features (Jabkowski & Kołczyńska, 2020). This documentation shall be appended after fieldwork with key information, such as the observed survey response rates, a description of any post-stratification, and the final weighting and variance estimation procedures (Gauthier et al., 2018).

Future Directions and Challenges

The work of GUIDE is not static. The most significant future challenge will be retention and attrition management. Maintaining participant engagement across two cohorts in many countries for decades will require constant innovation and significant, coordinated resources (see Chap. 10 in this book). Future directions will also involve adapting to new methodological opportunities, such as the integration of new administrative registers for sampling frames and adapting data collection strategies to new technologies. Rigorous documentation will be critical for this ongoing process, ensuring that future researchers can promote children's wellbeing growing up in digital Europe (see Chap. 1 in this book).

References

Anger, S., Laible, M., Trahms, A., & Vicari, B. (2019). Surveying lifelong learning in the German National Educational Panel Study. *Australian Economic Review, 52*(3), 353–362. https://doi.org/10.1111/1467-8462.12332

Bergmann, M., Kneip, T., De Luca, G., & Scherpenzeel, A. (2017). Survey participation in the survey of health. In *Ageing and retirement in Europe (SHARE), wave 1–6 (SHARE working paper series 31–2017)*. Economics of Aging (MEA).

Bergmann, M., & Scherpenzeel, A. (2016). Can a responsive fieldwork design increase response rates and decrease response bias in the Survey of Health, Ageing and Retirement in Europe. *SHARE Working Paper Series 27–2016*. Munich: Munich Center for the Economics of Aging (MEA).

Blöss, T. (2009). Travail domestique et responsabilités parentales: Présupposés et paradoxes de l'action publique. *Informations Sociales, 154*(4), 50–59. https://doi.org/10.3917/inso.154.0050

Carfagna, E., & Carfagna, A. (2015). Combining list frames with different kinds of area frame. In *60th ISI world statistics congress proceedings* (pp. 1–6).

Charles, M. A., Thierry, X., Lanoe, J.-L., Bois, C., Dufourg, M.-N., Popa, R., Cheminat, M., Zaros, C., & Geay, B. (2020). Cohort profile: The French national cohort of children (ELFE): Birth to 5 years. *International Journal of Epidemiology, 49*(2), 368–369. https://doi.org/10.1093/ije/dyz227

Couper, M. P., & Ofstedal, M. B. (2009). Keeping in contact with mobile sample members. In P. Lynn (Ed.), *Methodology of longitudinal surveys* (pp. 183–203). Wiley. https://doi.org/10.1002/9780470743874.ch11

De Luca, G., Rossetti, C., & Malter, F. (2015). Sample design and weighting strategies in SHARE Wave 5. In F. Malter & A. Börsch-Supan (Eds.), *SHARE Wave 5: Innovations & methodology* (pp. 75–84). Munich Center for the Economics of Aging (MEA).

Eckman, S., Himelein, K., & Dever, J. A. (2018). Innovative sample designs using GIS technology. In T. P. Johnson, B.-E. Pennell, I. A. L. Stoop, & B. Dorer (Eds.), *Advances in comparative survey methods: Multinational, multiregional, and multicultural contexts (3MC)* (pp. 67–92). Wiley.

ELFE. (2025). ELFE—Questionnaires and other useful documents. https://www.elfe-france.fr/en/cote-recherche/acces-aux-donnees-et-questionnaires/questionnaires-et-autres-documents

Eurostat. (2023). *Methodological guidelines and description of EU-SILC target variables*. https://ec.europa.eu/eurostat/documents/203647/20298610/Methodological+guidelines+2023+operation_v6-accessibility.pdf/2d6aa68c-aa51-d386-1f1c-0206fda5be49?t=1730709878443

Fokkema, T., Kveder, A., Hiekel, N., Emery, T., & Liefbroer, A. C. (2016). Generations and gender Programme wave 1 data collection: An overview and assessment of sampling and fieldwork methods, weighting procedures, and cross-sectional representativeness. *Demographic Research, 34*, 499–524. https://doi.org/10.4054/DemRes.2016.34.18

Gauthier, A. H., Cabaço, S. L. F., & Emery, T. (2018). Generations and gender survey study profile. *Longitudinal and Life Course Studies, 9*(4), 456–465. https://doi.org/10.14301/llcs.v9i4.500

Groves, R. M., Fowler Jr., F. J., Couper, M. P., Lepkowski, J. M., Singer, E., & Tourangeau, R. (2011). *Survey methodology* (2nd ed.). Wiley.

Groves, R. M., & Heeringa, S. G. (2006). Responsive design for household surveys: Tools for actively controlling survey errors and costs. *Journal of the Royal Statistical Society: Series A (Statistics in Society), 169*(3), 439–457. https://doi.org/10.1111/j.1467-985X.2006.00423.x

Häder, S., Gabler, S., Laaksonen, S., Lynn, P., & Purdon, S. (2003). *Final report: Sampling for the European social survey*. Norwegian Social Science Data Services.

Heeringa, S. G., & O'Muircheartaigh, C. (2010). Sample design for cross-cultural and cross-national survey programs. In J. A. Harkness, M. Braun, B. Edwards, T. P. Johnson, L. E. Lyberg, P. P. Mohler, B.-E. Pennell, & T. W. Smith (Eds.), *Survey methods in multinational, multiregional, and multicultural contexts* (pp. 251–267). Wiley.

Hubbard, F., Lin, Y., Zahs, D., & Hu, M. (2016). *Sample design*. Institute for Social Research, University of Michigan. http://ccsg.isr.umich.edu/

Iqbal, J. M., Faizan, D., & Mansha, G. (2018). A review on the recent development on the cluster sampling. *Biostatistics and Biometrics Open Access Journal, 5*(5), 555673. https://doi.org/10.19080/BBOAJ.2018.05.555673

Jabkowski, P., & Kołczyńska, M. (2020). Sampling and fieldwork practices in Europe: Analysis of methodological documentation from 1, 537 surveys in five cross-national projects, 1981–2017. *Methodology, 16*(3), 186–207. https://doi.org/10.5964/meth.2795

Jensen, A. L. (1991). Relative precision of stratified sampling, sampling with probability of selection proportional to size, and simple random sampling with ratio estimation. *Environmetrics, 2*(4), 475–486. https://doi.org/10.1002/env.3770020406

Kalton, G. (2023). Probability vs. nonprobability sampling: From the birth of survey sampling to the present day. *Statistics in Transition New Series, 24*(3), 1–22. https://doi.org/10.59170/stattrans-2023-029

Kreuter, F. (Ed.) (2013). *Improving surveys with paradata: Analytic uses of process information*. John Wiley & Sons. https://doi.org/10.1002/9781118596869

Lynn, P. (Ed.). (2009). *Methodology of longitudinal surveys*. John Wiley & Sons. https://doi.org/10.1002/9780470743874

Lynn, P. (2020). Methods for recruitment and retention (Understanding Society Working Paper No. 2020–07). University of Essex.

Lynn, P., Häder, S., Gabler, S., & Laaksonen, S. (2007). Methods for achieving equivalence of samples in cross-national surveys: The European social survey experience. *Journal of Official Statistics, 23*(1), 107–124.

Magnus, P., Birke, C., Vejrup, K., Haugan, A., Alsaker, E., Daltveit, A. K., Handal, M., Haugen, M., Høiseth, G., Knudsen, G. P., Paltiel, L., Schreuder, P., Tambs, K., Vold, L., & Stoltenberg, C. (2016). Cohort profile update: The Norwegian mother and child cohort study (MoBa). *International Journal of Epidemiology, 45*(2), 382–388. https://doi.org/10.1093/ije/dyw029

Magnus, P., Irgens, L. M., Haug, K., Nystad, W., Skjærven, R., & Stoltenberg, C. (2006). Cohort profile: The Norwegian mother and child cohort study (MoBa). *International Journal of Epidemiology, 35*(5), 1146–1150. https://doi.org/10.1093/ije/dyl170

Mazen, J. A. M., Tong, X., & Taylor, L. K. (2019). Evaluation of supplemental samples in longitudinal research with non-normal missing data. *Behavior Research Methods, 51*(3), 1321–1335. https://doi.org/10.3758/s13428-018-1070-3

MoBa. (2025). Protocols for the Norwegian mother, *Father and Child Cohort Study (MoBa)*. Norwegian Institute of Public Health. https://www.fhi.no/en/publ/2012/protocols-for-moba/

Neyman, J. (1992). On the two different aspects of the representative method: The method of stratified sampling and the method of purposive selection. In S. Kotz & N. L. Johnson (Eds.), *Breakthroughs in statistics: Methodology and distribution* (pp. 123–150). Springer.

Pace, D. S. (2021). Probability and non-probability sampling—An entry point for undergraduate researchers. *International Journal of Quantitative and Qualitative Research Methods, 9*(2), 1–15. https://www.eajournals.org/wp-content/uploads/Probability-and-Non-Probability-Sampling-an-entry-point-for-undergraduate-researchers

Pirus, C., Bois, C., Dufourg, M.-N., Lanoë, J.-L., Vandentorren, S., & Leridon, H. (2010). Constructing a cohort: Experience with the French ELFE project. *Population (English Edition), 65*(4), 543–567. https://doi.org/10.3917/pope.1004.0543

Quail, A., Williams, J., McCrory, C., Murray, A., & Thornton, M. (2011, April). Sample design and response in wave 1 of the infant cohort (at 9 months) of growing up in Ireland. *The Economic and Social Research Institute.*. https://www.growingup.gov.ie/pubs/SAMPLE-DESIGN-AND-RESPONSE-INFANTS.pdf

Schaeper, H. (2013). The German National Educational Panel Study (NEPS). In S. Blömeke, O. Zlatkin-Troitschanskaia, C. Kuhn, & J. Fege (Eds.), *Modeling and measuring competencies in higher education* (pp. 147–158). SensePublishers. https://doi.org/10.1007/978-94-6091-867-4_11

Scherpenzeel, A., Maineri, A., Bristle, J., Pflüger, S.-M., Mindarova, I., Butt, S., Zins, S., Emery, T., & Luijkx, R. (2017). *Report on the use of sampling frames in European studies*. SERISS.

Simard, M., & Franklin, S. (2005). Sample design guidelines. In *Generations and Gender Programme: Survey instruments* (pp. 5–14). United Nations Economic Commission for Europe. https://unece.org/DAM/pau/_docs/ggp/2005/GGP_2005_Publ.pdf

Smith, T. W. (2018). Improving multinational, multiregional, and multicultural (3MC) comparability using the total survey error (TSE) paradigm. In T. P. Johnson, B.-E. Pennell, I. A. L. Stoop, & B. Dorer (Eds.), *Advances in comparative survey methods: Multinational, multiregional, and multicultural contexts (3MC)* (pp. 13–43). Wiley.

Smith, P., Lynn, P., & Elliot, D. (2009). Sample design for longitudinal surveys. In P. Lynn (Ed.), *Methodology of longitudinal surveys* (pp. 21–33). Wiley. https://doi.org/10.1002/9780470743874.ch2

Survey Research Center. (2010). Guidelines for best practice in cross-cultural surveys. Survey Research Center, Institute for Social Research, University of Michigan. http://www.ccsg.isr.umich.edu/wp-content/uloads/2020/02/CCSG_Guidelines_Archive_2010_Version.pdf

Taylor, L. K., Tong, X., & Maxwell, S. E. (2020). Evaluating supplemental samples in longitudinal research: Replacement and refreshment approaches. *Multivariate Behavioral Research, 55*(2), 277–299. https://doi.org/10.1080/00273171.2019.1628694

Tourangeau, R., Brick, J. M., Lohr, S., & Li, J. (2017). Adaptive and responsive survey designs: A review and assessment. *Journal of the Royal Statistical Society: Series A (Statistics in Society), 180*(1), 203–223. https://doi.org/10.1111/rssa.12186

Valliant, R., Dever, J. A., & Kreuter, F. (2013). *Practical tools for designing and weighting survey samples*. Springer.

Zinn, S., Würbach, A., Steinhauer, H. W., & Hammon, A. (2020). Attrition and selectivity of the NEPS starting cohorts: An overview of the past 8 years. *AStA Wirtschafts- und Sozialstatistisches Archiv, 14*(2), 163–206. https://doi.org/10.1007/s11943-020-00268-7

Gaspar Massiot (Ph.D.) is a researcher in applied statistics associated with the French Institute for Demographic Studies (INED). He is in charge of the Sampling and Panel design of the Horizon Europe research project Growing Up in Digital Europe Preparation Phase (GUIDEPREP).

Shuang Su (Ph.D.) is a postdoctoral fellow at the School of Education, University College Dublin. Having obtained her Ph.D. in 2024, she specializes in digital wellbeing through mixed-methods research. She is currently working on the Horizon Europe research project Growing Up in Digital Europe Preparation Phase (GUIDEPREP).

Chapter 5
Developing a Cross-National, Longitudinal Questionnaire to Study Child Wellbeing

Toni Babarović, Eta Krpanec, Mirta Blažev, and Iva Černja Rajter

Introduction to Measuring Children and Youth Wellbeing

Children's and youth's wellbeing is crucial for their lives and positive development (Ben-Arieh et al., 2014). To gain a comprehensive understanding of the wellbeing of children and youth, it is crucial to evaluate it across various life domains, utilize multiple indicators, and recognize its dynamic nature (Axford et al., 2014; Cho & Yu, 2020; Goswami et al., 2016). Therefore, GUIDE takes a longitudinal, cross-national, and multidisciplinary approach to wellbeing, using a diverse set of measures and emphasizing a child-centered perspective. Such an ambitious approach presents challenges in achieving key objectives: valid, accurately translated, and culturally appropriate measurement; the need to encompass a wide range of topics; and the requirement for conciseness to maintain participant engagement. The following chapter presents the conceptualization, development, and the multi-step piloting process of GUIDE's survey on child wellbeing.

GUIDE's Approach to Questionnaire Development

Operationalization of the GUIDE Model of Child Wellbeing

GUIDE is designed as a longitudinal survey, including three core questionnaires for 8-year-old children, their parents and caregivers, and the parents and caregivers of infants. Questionnaire development was guided by a set of jointly agreed-upon assumptions among research partners, ensuring a comprehensive, theoretically

T. Babarović (✉) · E. Krpanec · M. Blažev · I. Č. Rajter
Ivo Pilar Institute of Social Sciences, Zagreb, Croatia
e-mail: toni.babarovic@pilar.hr

L. K. Taylor et al. (eds.), *Growing Up in Digital Europe*, Springer Series on Child and Family Studies, https://doi.org/10.1007/978-3-032-30592-3_5

grounded, and methodologically robust approach to measuring child wellbeing. The questionnaire development team strived to: identify the most relevant and comprehensive theoretical frameworks of child and youth wellbeing while differentiating between various conceptualizations of wellbeing found in previous research; capture all relevant aspects of wellbeing within a longitudinal framework, allowing for a deeper understanding of how wellbeing evolves; ensure that the study could provide comprehensible and relevant longitudinal data to inform diverse policymakers; and ensure that the data collected was scientifically rigorous, methodologically sound, and policy-relevant while also being organizationally and financially feasible for long-term implementation.

GUIDE's Wellbeing Model (see Chap. 1 in this book) integrates subjective and functional aspects of wellbeing while accounting for social and environmental influences. Its operationalization is structured around multiple interrelated dimensions that ensure a comprehensive and holistic understanding of child development: at the individual level, it includes children's emotional states, life satisfaction, autonomy, and functioning across cognitive, social, physical, and emotional domains; at the proximal level, it reflects environmental contexts such as home, school, neighborhoods, and digital access, as well as relationships with parents, teachers, and peers; and at the macrosystemic level, broader structural and policy-related factors—such as education, housing, and health systems—are incorporated using external data sources.

Methodological Foundations of GUIDE's Questionnaire Development

Building on the operationalization of the conceptual model, the GUIDE team started the process of developing the questionnaire. A core principle of questionnaire development was the adoption and adaptation of reliable and valid measurement instruments. Wherever possible, the research team prioritized well-established, empirically validated, and cross-culturally invariant instruments and scales. These selected instruments needed to be age-appropriate for respondents across the first and subsequent waves of data collection, ensuring that questions remained developmentally suitable over time. To maintain feasibility, the questionnaires were designed to be concise yet comprehensive, ensuring that they were ethically appropriate for face-to-face interviews and accessible for research purposes, whether publicly available or obtainable upon request (see Chap. 2 in this book). In cases where no suitable standardized instruments were available, new scales and survey items were developed through collaborative cross-cultural efforts among piloting teams. The proposed questionnaire underwent multiple, iterative rounds of refinement based on feedback from various stakeholders, including Youth Advisory Boards, to improve its clarity, validity, and usability.

Youth Advisory Board Recommendations for Questionnaire Development

Role of Youth Advisory Boards in the Questionnaire Development

In complex research projects and infrastructures, the perspectives of children and young people are often overlooked due to the perceived complexity of the research process and a prioritization of scientific objectives over participatory approaches (Cuevas-Parra & Tisdall, 2019). GUIDE is built on the principle that young people, as experts in their own lives, must have a voice in research that affects them. Previous studies have demonstrated that children and young people can meaningfully contribute to research, from the initial conceptualization to the design and implementation of research methodologies (Cuevas-Parra & Tisdall, 2019; Ramaj & Pollock, 2025). Their input improves the coherence, effectiveness, and child-friendliness of research materials, methodologies, and approaches, ultimately strengthening research rigor (Ramaj & Pollock, 2025). Children as active participants and advisors provide authentic insights that adults may overlook, making research findings more relevant, applicable, and reflective of their lived realities (Cuevas-Parra & Tisdall, 2019).

Recognizing this, the Youth Advisory Boards (YABs) were established as a consultative body to provide structured guidance on research concerning children and young people, as well as to support the development of the GUIDE questionnaire. These boards were formed in four European countries: Finland, Croatia, England, and Portugal. The YABs were purposefully designed not as representative structures in the traditional sense; rather, they aimed for diverse representation by recruiting young advisors from varied backgrounds—considering ethnicity, religion, socioeconomic status, culture, and ensuring balanced gender and age distribution. This diversity enabled the YABs to provide feedback informed by a wide range of perspectives, helping to ensure that study procedures and questionnaire content were inclusive, accessible, and developmentally appropriate. The target size was 2 to 6 members per country, with oversampling to account for potential attrition. Moreover, at least two members per country were proficient in English to facilitate cross-national collaboration.

The primary mission of the YABs was to ensure that GUIDE is child-centered and incorporates the perspectives of children and young people from the earliest stages of project design. By actively involving young people from diverse backgrounds and countries, the YABs promote a deeper understanding of the unique challenges and perspectives associated with research involving children and young people. This approach ensures that their lived experiences and diverse viewpoints are incorporated into the project processes, leading to research outcomes that are more inclusive, relevant, and reflective of the needs of the target population.

Within GUIDE, the YABs were instrumental in designing, piloting, and refining research methodologies and outputs, addressing areas such as ethical considerations, research tool development, and dissemination activities. Consultations with the YABs were carried out both nationally and internationally. Nationally, YABs convened one to two times per year to oversee, review, and advise researchers on key questions regarding project and joint research activities (COORDINATE, n.d.). Their contributions included engaging as stakeholders in ethical discussions, providing insights into research tool development, and reviewing essential materials such as training materials, questionnaires, and fieldwork procedures (see Chap. 3 in this book). Representatives from each national YAB met virtually at least twice, forming an International YAB. This crucial cross-national collaboration integrated diverse cultural and geographical perspectives, creating a unified platform for young advisors to share insights and enriching GUIDE's scope. Such cross-national collaboration was crucial for integrating diverse cultural perspectives and creating a unified platform for young advisors to share insights across countries (COORDINATE, 2023).

Youth Advisory Board's Feedback on GUIDE Questionnaire Content and Study Procedures

YABs across Finland and Croatia were particularly involved in reviewing GUIDE procedures and questionnaire development through a series of three workshops conducted in 2022. These workshops were essential for integrating youth advisors' perspectives and making necessary adjustments to the study design, ensuring that research instruments and procedures were both child-friendly and methodologically rigorous. The primary objectives of the workshops were to gather feedback on study procedures and questionnaire content while also exploring improvements for future research rounds.

The first workshop introduced young advisors to GUIDE, familiarizing them with its objectives, questionnaire content, and procedural elements. Discussions emphasized the importance of pilot studies in identifying potential methodological challenges before the main research phase. Young advisors provided recommendations on several critical aspects, including the optimal duration and location of interviews, strategies for rapport-building, the role of parents and caregivers during interviews, and appropriate incentives to encourage participation. These suggestions were essential in shaping the GUIDE pilot study, as they aimed to foster a supportive and comfortable environment for younger participants, ensuring their active engagement and overall wellbeing.

The second workshop focused on an in-depth review of the GUIDE questionnaire, as young advisors self-completed the survey and assessed its clarity, relevance, and appropriateness, particularly for younger children. Their feedback highlighted the need to simplify complex questions, eliminate redundancies, shorten the questionnaire, and prioritize themes most relevant to children and young people.

These refinements helped ensure that the questionnaire was accessible, engaging, and developmentally appropriate, ultimately improving data quality and response reliability.

In the third workshop, young advisors evaluated the feasibility of administering the GUIDE questionnaire to children as young as eight years old. They emphasized the importance of adapting the questionnaire to align with the attention spans and comprehension levels of younger participants. Their recommendations included child-friendly interview processes, such as casual introductions, rapport-building activities, and small incentives to foster trust and comfort. Additionally, young advisors stressed the importance of conducting interviews in secure and familiar environments (e.g., homes or school libraries) while avoiding the presence of parents and caregivers to minimize potential biases. These insights were crucial in ensuring ethical and effective engagement with younger participants.

The YAB workshops demonstrated the value of involving young people in research design and methodological development. By incorporating the YAB's feedback into the further development of study procedures and the questionnaire, GUIDE's tools and procedures were significantly improved, becoming more accessible, relevant, and effective for the target population, ultimately contributing to more robust questionnaire development.

Questionnaire Description

Construction of the Questionnaires

Based on the conceptual model and feedback from the youth advisory boards, we proposed a version of a questionnaire for 8-year-old children, a questionnaire for their parents and caregivers, and a questionnaire for the parents and caregivers of infants. The two questionnaires developed for parents and caregivers share a core set of questions, supplemented by additional age-appropriate questions. In the proposed versions of the questionnaires, some of the items were constructed by the research team, but the majority were adopted from well-known and previously validated scales. A detailed overview of questionnaire modules and themes can be found in the tables (see Tables 5.1 and 5.2).

Response categories for questions in all questionnaires were in the form of words, numbers, or scales. For certain questions, showcards—visual aids displaying the answer categories on the electronic screen—were used to reduce the cognitive burden on participants and improve response accuracy. Both child and caregiver questionnaires conclude with the evaluation of the questionnaire and interviewing process and interviewers' observations regarding the interviewing process.

All data were planned to be collected either face-to-face or via video with Computer-Assisted Personal Interviewing (CAPI). This primary method was supplemented by a self-completion questionnaire for parents and caregivers (see Chap. 3

Table 5.1 Children's questionnaire

Module	Themes
Socio-demographic data and filter questions	– Gender – Age – Grade – Type of schooling – Access to electronic devices and internet
Rapport and confidence building	– Introductory questions
Hedonic wellbeing	– Life satisfaction – Positive and negative affect – Safety
Eudaimonic wellbeing	– Meaning and purpose – Basic psychological needs satisfaction – Self-acceptance/self-esteem – Voice
Physical functioning	– General and specific physical functioning – Body image
Emotional functioning	– Emotional reappraisal – Internalized and externalized emotional problems
Social functioning	– Prosocial behavior
Cognitive functioning	– Academic functioning
School	– School satisfaction – Teacher and student support
Family	– Parental relationship with the main and the other caregiver – Home life satisfaction – Care for family members
Friends	– Satisfaction with friendship
Bullying	– Bullying victim and perpetrator
Leisure activities	– Participation in organized and unorganized leisure activities
Digital	– School day and weekend digital use – Digital activities – Parental monitoring – Digital addiction and enjoyment
Material	– Financial resources and family stress
Neighborhood	

in this book). This self-completion format was reserved for questions evaluated as sensitive, including those regarding pregnancy, relationship with the child, relationship with non-resident biological parent and/or current relationship, satisfaction with different aspects of life, parental stress and mental wellbeing, and so on.

Table 5.2 Parents and caregiver questionnaire

Module	Parents and caregivers of infants: themes	Parents and caregivers of 8-year-olds: themes
Household information	– Main caregiver and child – Other household members	– Main caregiver and child – Other household members
Socio-demographic data	– Marital and relationship status – Nationality and citizenship	– Marital and relationship status – Nationality and citizenship
Employment and socio-economic conditions	– Employment and education – Economic hardship and income	– Employment and education – Economic hardship and income
Housing, neighborhood, and community	– Housing and accommodation – Neighborhood and community	– Housing and accommodation – Neighborhood and community
Pregnancy and birth	– Pregnancy and prenatal care – Delivery and physical development at birth	– Pregnancy and prenatal care – Delivery and physical development at birth
Child's health and wellbeing	– Child's diet – Child's health and use of health services	– Child's diet – Child's health and use of health services – Child's emotional health and wellbeing
Child's education	N/A	– Child's school – Learning difficulties – Parental involvement
Child's activities	N/A	– Child's activities and leisure – Electronic devices
Parenting	N/A	– Parenting practices – Parenting activities and behaviors – Family cohesion
Child's development and habits	– Child's development – Child's skills and habits	N/A
Childcare	– Childcare arrangements – Support or help from others	– Childcare arrangements
Child's functioning and relationships	– Child's functioning and relationships	N/A

(continued)

Table 5.2 (continued)

Module	Parents and caregivers of infants: themes	Parents and caregivers of 8-year-olds: themes
Respondent's and family health	– General health – Physical or mental health problems	– General health – Physical or mental health problems
Self-completion	– Relationship with non-resident biological parent – Satisfaction with current relationship – Satisfaction with different aspects of life and parental stress – Information about the pregnancy with the child	– Relationship with non-resident biological parent – Satisfaction with current relationship – Satisfaction with different aspects of life and parental stress – Information about the pregnancy with the child – Bullying

Questionnaire Translation

Overview of the TRAPD Methodology

The survey questionnaires, interviewer guides, and CAPI software were translated from English to the official languages of the countries where the pilot is going to be carried out: Croatian, French, Finnish, and Slovenian. The translation of the survey questionnaires was done following the Translation, Review, Adjudication, Pretesting, Documentation (TRAPD) methodology, which is widely regarded as a best practice for ensuring high-quality and comparable translations in multinational survey research (Harkness et al., 2010; Willis et al., 2010). This methodology, implemented by each national partner, involves a systematic and iterative process including five phases that ensure linguistic, cultural, and conceptual accuracy while maintaining comparability across the various language versions of the survey instruments (see Chap. 9 in this book).

In the *Translation* phase, translators create the initial version of the text using clear instructions based on the study's goals. In the *Review* phase, bilingual experts evaluate the translation to identify issues and suggest improvements. In the *Adjudication* phase, a decision-maker or small group evaluates these suggestions, resolves any discrepancies identified during the review, and finalizes the translation, ensuring it is both accurate and culturally appropriate. The *Pretesting* phase uses methods such as cognitive interviews and pilot testing to assess the translation and make improvements based on respondents' feedback. Finally, the *Documentation* phase involves recording all decisions made and issues that arose during each phase, ensuring the entire process is transparent and can be reviewed or traced if needed (Harkness et al., 2010; Willis et al., 2010).

In sum, the TRAPD methodology is particularly suited for complex multinational projects, as it emphasizes team-based collaboration and continuous adjustments at every stage of the translation process. This approach ensures that translations are both accurate and culturally appropriate, making it an essential tool for projects like GUIDE, which involve multiple partners from diverse cultural and linguistic backgrounds.

Tools and Processes for Translation and Quality Assurance

Partners followed the TRAPD procedure with the support of an online software platform. The platform was designed to streamline and coordinate the translation process within national teams, allowing the central team to oversee their work, while systematically storing and reporting structured information at each phase of the translation process (e.g., draft translations, comments, final translation).

To ensure high-quality and linguistically robust translations, GUIDE complemented the TRAPD process with targeted involvement of specialized linguistic quality assurance (LQA) experts. These professionals did not perform all TRAPD roles (i.e., Translator, Reviewer, Adjudicator, Pretester, and Documenter) but were instead engaged in specific phases—primarily review and adjudication—to independently assess translatability, address cultural nuances, and ensure linguistic consistency. Their focused involvement provided a final layer of quality control before pretesting and final deployment, while significantly enhancing translation accuracy and cross-language harmonization (Behr, 2018; Harkness et al., 2010; ISO 17100, 2015). For GUIDE, experts at cApStAn, a prominent language service provider specializing in LQA for multilingual research (cApStAn, n.d.), conducted an in-depth assessment of the questionnaires. Their assessment focused on detecting linguistic ambiguities, ensuring cultural appropriateness, and identifying potential translatability challenges. Their approach follows internationally recognized standards, including the International Test Commission's Guidelines for Translating and Adapting Tests (ITC, 2017) and the University of Michigan's Cross-Cultural Survey Guidelines (Survey Research Center, 2016). As a result of this rigorous quality control, several refinements and improvements were introduced into the GUIDE questionnaire, improving its clarity, accuracy, and cross-language consistency. Engaging LQA specialists like those at cApStAn in multinational projects, such as GUIDE, has proven to be a valuable strategic approach for achieving high-quality, culturally relevant, and internationally comparable translations.

Piloting GUIDE Questionnaires

Definition and Importance of Piloting

Although definitions of piloting vary among researchers, certain core elements are shared: a pilot occurs before the main study, operates on a smaller scale, and aims to refine the main study's design and feasibility. Definitions from scholars such as Porta (2008) and Polit et al. (2001) emphasize piloting as a preparatory phase to test methods, instruments, or protocols. The pilot process helps researchers identify potential failures or weaknesses in the study design, refine instruments, and evaluate feasibility without expending unnecessary resources. For large, resource-intensive studies, piloting is not just a useful tool but an essential step in the research process.

Types of Pilots

Previous research provided a systematic and comprehensive overview of common approaches and best practices for piloting in birth-cohort longitudinal studies (Blažev et al., 2021). This includes identifying the main types of pilot studies, their sampling strategies, and how frequently pilots are conducted in preparation for the main study (Blažev et al., 2021). This research highlighted the importance of thorough documentation to ensure pilot studies are both replicable and informative.

Three types of pilot studies are typically used before each wave of the main study: pre-pilots, instrument pilots, and dress rehearsals (Blažev et al., 2021). Each type has a distinct objective, is conducted at a different stage of study preparations, and employs distinct methods (Blažev et al., 2021).

- *Pre-pilots* are small-scale exploratory studies, typically involving 8–50 participants, designed to explore and refine study instruments during the early phases of research. These often involve qualitative methods, such as in-depth interviews, to guide the development of questionnaires and study protocols.
- *Instrument pilots* are medium-sized studies, involving up to 350 participants, focusing on testing the design and content of the research instruments. This phase ensures the validity and reliability of questionnaires by assessing their structure, content, and psychometric properties.
- *Dress rehearsals* are large-scale trials, with up to 1500 participants, designed to simulate the full implementation of the study. This phase evaluates all fieldwork processes, including recruitment strategies, data collection methods, and operational procedures, to identify and resolve potential issues before the main study begins.

Each type of pilot study is tailored to the specific needs of the research, contributing to the overall quality and reliability of longitudinal birth cohort studies.

Piloting in GUIDE

While designing and implementing piloting procedures for GUIDE, we relied on the above-mentioned findings by Blažev et al. (2021) regarding piloting in the field of large, longitudinal birth cohort studies. We employed a multi-step piloting approach, comprising a pre-pilot, which utilized cognitive interviews, and an instrument pilot, which evaluated the psychometric properties of the questionnaires. For GUIDE, a dress rehearsal is planned in the next period to simulate the full research process. All the piloting procedures were done cross-nationally with both child and carer participants to ensure appropriateness of the questionnaire across samples.

GUIDE Pre-pilot: Cognitive Interviews

Cognitive Interviewing Methodology

Pre-piloting of GUIDE questionnaire items included cognitive interviews, which evaluate whether survey questions meet their goals by analyzing respondents' thought processes (see Chap. 6 in this book; Collins, 2015). Cognitive interviews were conducted on 68 8-year-old children and 40 parents and caregivers of those children or infants across Croatia (20 children, 10 parents and caregivers), France (18 children, 10 parents and caregivers), Finland (10 children, 10 parents and caregivers), and Ireland (20 children, 10 parents and caregivers). Child interviews addressed wellbeing through 31 items split into two subsamples, while carer questionnaires covered 37 items. Items that were evaluated as most difficult or problematic were chosen to be included in the cognitive interviews. Interviews were conducted in-person or remotely via video call, with written consent obtained. Data was analyzed by national teams and cross-national experts.

Key Findings and Recommendations from Child and Carer Interviews

Cognitive interviewing yielded important implications for questionnaire design. The detailed findings of the cognitive interview were published in a paper by Babarović et al. (2024). In sum, the results of the children interviews suggested creating a safe environment for children, training interviewers, and reconsidering complex questions. Simplifying language, using child-friendly examples, and avoiding abstract timeframes or mean-value estimates were emphasized. Likert scales were suitable but required clear neutral descriptors and minimal variation. Caregiver interviews prompted several rounds of refinement, beginning with minor changes focused on clarifying terms and improving question flow. More substantial changes included adapting culturally specific response categories while maintaining cross-cultural comparability. Recall questions were changed from open-ended to closed-ended formats, and sensitive questions were changed to self-completion modules. General recommendations included harmonizing child and carer questionnaires for comparability, using filters to reduce burden, and ensuring adaptable formats for diverse cultural contexts.

GUIDE Instrument Pilot

Instrument Piloting Across Five European Countries

GUIDE's instrument piloting used a harmonized research design across five European countries: Croatia, Finland, France, Ireland, and Slovenia. Scientific teams collaborated with Ipsos and Kantar agencies, with support from the GUIDE Central Hub and Center data. The preparation phase included selecting agencies, designing and translating questionnaires, obtaining ethical approvals, and training interviewers. Fieldwork was focused on piloting questionnaires for 8-year-old children, their parents and caregivers, and parents and caregivers of infants. Each country targeted 250 respondents per group, except for Finland (167 respondents per group, due to budget limits). Surveys primarily used face-to-face, CAPI interviews, with Finland employing CAVI (Computer-Assisted Video Interviewing). Recruitment methods varied, with most countries offering financial incentives.

Key Insights from Fieldwork and Questionnaire Analysis

We analyzed two aspects of the pilot instrument: fieldwork and questionnaires. The fieldwork analysis included an assessment of recruitment and sample characteristics, fieldwork and data storage procedures (see Chap. 3 in this book), as well as the analysis of feedback from participants and interviewers. The questionnaire analysis focused on the psychometric properties of the used items and scales.

The results of the fieldwork analysis provided valuable recommendations for future fieldwork procedures. In terms of recruitment, the analysis indicated that using financial incentives could increase interest and satisfaction with participation in the study. For example, French participants, who did not receive financial incentives, reported lower interest and a reduced likelihood of future participation than their counterparts from other countries. In addition to the observed usefulness of financial incentives, other strategies that helped the recruitment were utilizing existing panels rather than approaching possible participants in public and sending advance letters about the study. A level of familiarity with the study procedure and content seems to be pivotal for possible participants (Leeuw et al., 2007). However, providing information about the study should not be overdone, as it was reported that overly lengthy and complex consent forms discouraged participants from entering the research. An additional recruitment issue which was analyzed was the inclusion of hard-to-reach groups in the samples. It was concluded that the inclusion of recruiting via social media and using CAVI interviewing could encourage an increased number of participants from hard-to-reach groups (Forgasz et al., 2018; Thunberg & Arnell, 2021).

In terms of the interview procedure, the analysis suggested that using CAVI is a viable option, as Finnish participants rated it favorably in the evaluation of the study. Compared to the CAPI method, the CAVI method is less expensive and more convenient for the participants. However, transitioning to the CAVI method for interviewing children may not be feasible, as CAVI interview times for children were substantially longer than CAPI interviews and child participants from Finland did not provide very favorable assessments of their satisfaction with interviews.

Furthermore, the interviewer training sessions on working with children could be deepened or expanded upon. Many of the interviewers did not have prior experience interviewing children, which can pose specific challenges (Ponizovsky-Bergelson et al., 2019). Hence, there should be a more thorough preparation of the interviewers working with child participants.

The analysis of evaluations from interviewers and participants indicated general satisfaction with the interview process and content. However, a few notable recommendations were gathered. Interviewers reported that certain items seemed to be age-inappropriate for children, mainly ones considering meaning and purpose scales in the eudaimonic wellbeing section. Combined with psychometric analysis, which will be discussed in the next section, it was concluded that these scales were removed from the questionnaire or substantially revised. Additionally, evaluations suggested that the overall questionnaires were overly exhaustive. The participants felt some of the items were repetitive or lengthy. Thus, the items were reformulated to avoid exhaustiveness and redundancy. Hence, it is recommended that the questionnaires should strike a balance between reducing the number of items while ensuring the validity and reliability of the included scales. Furthermore, both participants and interviewers considered certain questions intrusive. This is problematic since intrusive questions tend to increase missing data and false reports (Tourangeau & Yan, 2007). Thus, it was assessed that more questions should be included in the self-competition module to encourage truthful answers. Finally, evaluations indicated a need for even greater emphasis on the translation process. While translation and cultural adaptation were detailed, some errors and places for improvement were noticed.

In addition to fieldwork analysis, we conducted a questionnaire analysis focused on the psychometric properties of each scale. Specifically, we performed a descriptive and non-response analysis on the item and scale level and assessed the reliability and structure of scales for each country sample. The analyses of both children's and parents and caregivers' questionnaires generally indicated the appropriateness of the items. Participants answered questions without difficulty, as the percentage of "I don't know" answers or refusals to answer did not surpass 3% on most items. The vast majority of scales had high reliability, expected one-factor structure, and satisfactory factor loadings (Hair et al., 2010; Kline, 2000).

A common issue with both children and carer questionnaires, consistent with the findings of fieldwork analysis, was that the questionnaires need to be shortened and that translation and cultural adaptation need to be improved. For example, the non-response analysis of certain more exhaustive and longer scales in the children questionnaire (e.g., leisure activities scale) indicated an increase in missing data for later items. Thus, the items were reformulated to avoid exhaustiveness and redundancy. The issues with translation and cultural adaptation were visible through worse psychometric properties or more non-responses to certain items only in some countries, rather than the overall sample. For instance, for some items and scales, there was a visible drop in response rate only in a specific sample, indicating that the question was problematic exclusively in that sample rather than overall. Each country's team was warned about these problematic items to improve them for the future study.

In terms of recommendations specific to the children's questionnaire, the analysis suggested a few areas for improvement. Primarily, the psychometric data provided support for fieldwork findings about the difficulties around certain items for children. Children had difficulties answering items of the meaning and purpose scale, emotional reappraisal scale, digital enjoyment scale, and financial resources and family stress scale, which was indicated by a surge in "I don't know" answers. Hence, these scales were either removed (e.g., meaning and purpose and emotional reappraisal scale) or significantly changed in the subsequent questionnaire version. Similarly, children had difficulties answering items that required them to take the perspectives of others (e.g., "Do the people who you like also like you?"); therefore, such items were reworded in a manner that is more focused on children's perspective (e.g., "Do you think that the people who you like also like you?"). Another issue in comprehension was found with items about digital device use. Contrary to our expectations, a large proportion of children answered that they do not use electronic devices (from 2.7% in Croatia, up to 19.5% in Slovenia). Out of those using electronic devices, many reported they are not allowed to use the Internet (from 3.2% in Croatia, up to 33.8% in France). Thus, it was concluded that these questions require additional review, as the results indicate that children may have misunderstood the question. Finally, children provided illogical answers to items with reverse scoring, resulting in lower reliability of scales that contained them. Thus, such items were rephrased or removed from the scales.

The analysis of the carer's questionnaire indicated a need for technical improvements, such as data entry and extraction processes. For instance, there should be a clearer procedure for coding country-specific answers, standardizing physical measurements across countries (e.g., weight in kilos or pounds), and introducing drop-down menus to minimize errors. In addition, it has been concluded that some of the items should be moved to a self-completion section or revised due to their sensitive nature. Items about pregnancy, socio-economic status, and health had an increased number of "I don't know" answers or refusals to answer due to being perceived as overly intimate.

Overall, instrument piloting provided valuable insights for future cross-national surveys and affirmed the GUIDE questionnaire's robust foundation for broader research.

Conclusions

Summary of Findings and Implications for GUIDE

The development and piloting of the GUIDE questionnaire have demonstrated the importance of meticulous design, cross-cultural adaptation, and thorough testing in creating questionnaires to assess children's wellbeing cross-nationally. By integrating validated scales, youth advisory board feedback, and culturally sensitive methodologies such as the TRAPD translation approach, the project ensured that the questionnaires are both scientifically robust and appropriate for diverse contexts. Multi-step pilots using a pre-pilot and an instrument pilot highlighted key adjustments needed for language clarity, cultural relevance, and participant comfort, particularly for younger respondents. These efforts have laid a solid foundation for the GUIDE questionnaire to advance research and policy focused on child wellbeing.

Future Steps in GUIDE Questionnaire Development

Before the beginning of GUIDE Wave 1 and throughout its 25-year duration, numerous aspects related to the development of questionnaires for children and their parents and caregivers will require ongoing attention. To prepare for GUIDE Wave 1, the questionnaires should undergo further translation and cultural adaptation across all participating countries, particularly those that did not take part in earlier piloting (i.e., Ireland, Finland, France, Croatia, and Slovenia). Following this, initial piloting of both the questionnaires and the interviewing procedures should be carried out in all participating countries. The final stage of pre-testing, a dress rehearsal, should then be conducted. This rehearsal serves to test recruitment, sampling, and fieldwork procedures for GUIDE, while also assessing the questionnaires on a broader scale than an instrument pilot (Blažev et al., 2021). Hence, in this step, we should be able to identify and proactively address practical challenges that may arise during GUIDE and pilot any final adaptations made in the questionnaires.

However, efforts to enhance the quality of measurements will not conclude with the initiation of GUIDE Wave 1. Given its 25-year timeline, continuous adjustments to the questionnaires will be necessary to account for the evolving needs and interests of the children as they grow, mature, and experience developmental changes (Zubrick, 2016). These adjustments must also respond to broader shifts in technology, policies, economic conditions, and social circumstances, which will impact the wellbeing of children and young people (Zubrick, 2016). The overarching objective of GUIDE is to remain responsive to these changes, ensuring the collection of meaningful and up-to-date data on the wellbeing of children and youth in the future. Therefore, ongoing consultations with Youth Advisory Boards and continuous piloting will be essential to maintaining the highest standards for the GUIDE questionnaires.

References

Axford, N., Jodrell, D., & Hobbs, T. (2014). Objective or subjective wellbeing? In A. Ben-Arieh, F. Casas, I. Frønes, & J. E. Korbin (Eds.), *Handbook of child wellbeing: Theories, methods and policies in global perspective* (pp. 1–28). Springer.

Babarović, T., Krpanec, E., Blažev, M., Dević, I., Downey, S., Huttunen, I., Panico, L., Perron, Z., Santos, A., Taylor, L. K., Upadyaya, K., Symonds, J., & Pollock, G. (2024). Children's understanding of wellbeing related questions: Results of cognitive interviews in four European countries. *International Journal of Social Research Methodology*. Advance online publication. https://doi.org/10.1080/13645579.2024.2312621

Behr, D. (2018). Translating questionnaires for cross-national surveys: A description of a genre and its particularities based on the ISO 17100 categorization of translator competences. *The International Journal for Translation & Interpreting Research, 10*(2), 1–16. https://doi.org/10.12807/ti.110202.2018.a02

Ben-Arieh, A., Casas, F., Frønes, I., & Korbin, J. E. (2014). Multifaceted concept of child wellbeing. In A. Ben-Arieh, F. Casas, I. Frønes, & J. E. Korbin (Eds.), *Handbook of child wellbeing: Theories, methods and policies in global perspective* (pp. 1–28). Springer.

Blažev, M., Babarović, T., & Serracant, P. (2021). Characteristics of piloting longitudinal birth cohort surveys: A systematic review. *Quality & Quantity, 55*(3), 1047–1069. https://doi.org/10.1007/s11135-020-01042-1

cApStAn. (n.d.). *Linguistic quality assurance*. cApStAn. https://www.capstan.be/linguistic-quality-assurance/

Casas, F., & Rees, G. (2015). Measures of children's subjective wellbeing: Analysis of the potential for cross-national comparisons. *Child Indicators Research, 8*(1), 49–69. https://doi.org/10.1007/s12187-014-9293-z

Cho, E. Y.-N., & Yu, F.-Y. (2020). A review of measurement tools for child wellbeing. *Children and Youth Services Review, 119*, Article 105576. https://doi.org/10.1016/j.childyouth.2020.105576

Cohen, J. F. W., Kraak, V. I., Choumenkovitch, S. F., Hyatt, R. R., & Economos, C. D. (2014). The CHANGE study: A healthy-lifestyles intervention to improve rural children's diet quality. *Journal of the Academy of Nutrition and Dietetics, 114*(1), 48–53. https://doi.org/10.1016/j.jand.2013.08.014

Collins, D. (2015). Cognitive interviewing: Origin, purpose and limitations. In D. Collins (Ed.), *Cognitive interviewing practice* (pp. 3–27). SAGE Publications. https://doi.org/10.4135/9781473910102

COORDINATE. (2023). *Children's wellbeing and rights: The role of longitudinal data* [Report]. COORDINATE Project. https://www.coordinate-network.eu/_files/ugd/90d31c_5185c4036b9c474d9491069c8cb8351a.pdf

COORDINATE. (n.d.). *Youth advisory board*. COORDINATE. https://www.coordinate-network.eu/youth-advisory-board

Cuevas-Parra, P., & Tisdall, E. K. M. (2019). Child-led research: Questioning knowledge. *Social Sciences, 8*(2), Article 44. https://doi.org/10.3390/socsci8020044

Driscoll, K., & Pianta, R. C. (2011). Mothers' and fathers' perceptions of conflict and closeness in parent-child relationships during early childhood. *Journal of Early Childhood and Infant Psychology, 7*, 1–24.

Forgasz, H., Tan, H., Leder, G., & McLeod, A. (2018). Enhancing survey participation: Facebook advertisements for recruitment in educational research. *International Journal of Research & Method in Education, 41*(3), 257–270. https://doi.org/10.1080/1743727X.2017.1295939

Goswami, H., Fox, C., & Pollock, G. (2016). The current evidence base and future needs in improving children's wellbeing across Europe: Is there a case for a comparative longitudinal survey? *Child Indicators Research, 9*, 371–388. https://doi.org/10.1007/s12187-015-9323-5

Hair, J. F., Black, W. C., Babin, B. J., & Anderson, R. E. (2010). *Multivariate data analysis* (7th ed.). Pearson.

Harkness, J. A., Villar, A., & Edwards, B. (2010). Translation, adaptation, and design. In J. A. Harkness, M. Braun, B. Edwards, T. P. Johnson, L. E. Lyberg, P. P. Mohler, B.-E. Pennell, & T. W. Smith (Eds.), *Survey methods in multinational, multiregional, and multicultural contexts* (pp. 115–140). John Wiley & Sons.

International Survey of Children's Well-Being (ISCWeB). (2018). *National reports*. Jacobs Foundation. https://isciweb.org/wp-content/uploads/2020/08/Childrens-Worlds-3rd-Wave-National-Reports-with-England.pdf

International Test Commission. (2017). *ITC guidelines for translating and adapting tests* (2nd ed.). https://www.intestcom.org/files/guideline_test_adaptation_2ed.pdf

International Organization for Standardization. (2015). *ISO 17100: Translation services—Requirements for translation services*. https://www.iso.org/obp/ui/#iso:std:iso:17100:ed-1:v1:en

Kline, P. (2000). *The handbook of psychological testing* (2nd ed.). Routledge.

Leeuw, E. D., Callegaro, M., Hox, J., Korendijk, E., & Lensvelt-Mulders, G. (2007). The influence of advance letters on response in telephone surveys: A meta-analysis. *Public Opinion Quarterly, 71*(3), 413–443. https://doi.org/10.1093/poq/nfm014

Mistry, R. S., Benner, A. D., Tan, C. S., & Kim, S. Y. (2009). Family economic stress and academic wellbeing among Chinese American youth: The influence of adolescents' perceptions of economic strain. *Journal of Family Psychology, 23*(3), 279–290. https://doi.org/10.1037/a0015403

Polit, D. F., Beck, C. T., & Hungler, B. P. (2001). *Essentials of nursing research: Methods, appraisal, and utilization* (5th ed.). Lippincott.

Porta, M. (2008). *A dictionary of epidemiology*. 5th ed. Oxford University Press.

Ponizovsky-Bergelson, Y., Dayan, Y., Wahle, N., & Roer-Strier, D. (2019). A qualitative interview with young children: What encourages or inhibits young children's participation? *International Journal of Qualitative Methods, 18*, 1–9. https://doi.org/10.1177/1609406919840516

Ramaj, K., & Pollock, G. (2025). Youth Advisory Boards (YABs): The case of Growing Up in Digital Europe (GUIDE). In E. Çela, E. Xhemi, F. Sipos, P. Krasztev, & Z. H. Bíró (Eds.), *Equity in education: A handbook for participative approaches in research and development to address school inequalities* (pp. 126–144). CEEOL Press. https://ceeolpress.com/book/35

Smahel, D., Machackova, H., Mascheroni, G., Dedkova, L., Staksrud, E., Ólafsson, K., Livingstone, S., & Hasebrink, U. (2020). *EU Kids Online 2020: Survey results from 19 countries*. EU Kids Online. https://doi.org/10.21953/lse.47fdeqj01ofo

Survey Research Center. (2016). *Guidelines for best practice in cross-cultural surveys* (4th ed.). Survey Research Center, Institute for Social Research, University of Michigan. https://ccsg.isr.umich.edu/wp-content/uploads/2019/06/CCSG_Full_Guidelines_2016_Version.pdf

Thunberg, S., & Arnell, L. (2021). Pioneering the use of technologies in qualitative research—A research review of the use of digital interviews. *International Journal of Social Research Methodology, 25*(6), 757–768. https://doi.org/10.1080/13645579.2021.1935565

Tourangeau, R., & Yan, T. (2007). Sensitive questions in surveys. *Psychological Bulletin, 133*(5), 859–883. https://doi.org/10.1037/0033-2909.133.5.859

Wespieser, K. (2015). *Young people and e-safety: The results of the 2015 London Grid for Learning e-safety survey*. National Foundation for Educational Research. https://files.eric.ed.gov/fulltext/ED558604.pdf

Willis, G. B., Kudela, M. S., Levin, K., Norberg, A., Stark, D. S., Forsyth, B. H., & Hartman, A. M. (2010). Evaluation of a multistep survey translation process. In J. A. Harkness, M. Braun, B. Edwards, T. P. Johnson, L. E. Lyberg, P. P. Mohler, B.-E. Pennell, & T. W. Smith (Eds.), *Survey methods in multinational, multiregional, and multicultural contexts* (pp. 141–167). John Wiley & Sons.

Zubrick, S. (2016). Longitudinal research: Applications for the design, conduct and dissemination of early childhood research. In A. Farrell, S. L. Kagan, & E. K. M. Tisdall (Eds.), *The SAGE handbook of early childhood research* (pp. 201–222). SAGE.

Toni Babarović (Ph.D.) is a professor at the Department of Psychology, University of Split, Croatia. His research focuses on educational psychology, particularly in areas such as career decision-making, school effectiveness, and educational management. He has contributed to various publications, including studies on career decision-making difficulties and the role of parents' beliefs in students' motivation and achievement.

Eta Krpanec (Ph.D.) is a research assistant at the Institute of Social Sciences Ivo Pilar in Croatia. She earned her Ph.D. in Psychology from the University of Zagreb. Her research focuses on educational psychology, particularly student agency, motivation, teaching styles, and the interrelationships between them.

Mirta Blažev (Ph.D.) is a research associate at the Institute of Social Sciences Ivo Pilar, Croatia, and an integrative psychotherapist. She holds a Ph.D. in Psychology and master's degrees in both Psychology and Economics. Her research addresses gender inequalities in education and the psychosocial challenges faced by youth.

Iva Černja Rajter (Ph.D.) is a postdoc at the Institute of Social Sciences Ivo Pilar and an assistant professor at the University of Zagreb. She earned her Ph.D. in 2022, specializes in career development, and is involved in several research projects, including Horizon Europe research project Growing Up in Digital Europe Preparation Phase (GUIDEPREP).

Chapter 6
Cognitive Assessment in Children

Iva Černja Rajter, Toni Babarović, and Ivan Dević

Introduction

Cognitive abilities are the mental processes through which children acquire knowledge and understanding of the world. They include processes such as memory, problem-solving, attention, and reasoning, which play a central role in learning and overall development (Sternberg, 2021). Cognitive abilities are crucial in childhood because they form the foundation for academic achievement, problem-solving throughout life, and social functioning. Assessing cognitive abilities enables both a developmental understanding of children and helps decide what interventions will be most beneficial (Flanagan & Harrison, 2012).

The aim of this chapter is to explore the methods and challenges of measuring cognitive abilities in children in the context of GUIDE, a longitudinal study aimed at understanding developmental trajectories across Europe. Focusing on traditional and nonverbal assessment methods, this chapter discusses appropriate measures of cognitive abilities in multicultural longitudinal studies. The article highlights how effective cognitive assessment can contribute to targeted interventions, development policies, and overall improvements in children's developmental outcomes. This chapter delves into various aspects of cognitive assessment, theoretical foundations, practical applications, and ethical considerations, highlighting how GUIDE offers a significant contribution to research and policy.

I. Č. Rajter (✉) · T. Babarović · I. Dević
Institute of Social Sciences Ivo Pilar, Zagreb, Croatia
e-mail: icernja@pilar.hr

L. K. Taylor et al. (eds.), *Growing Up in Digital Europe*, Springer Series on Child and Family Studies, https://doi.org/10.1007/978-3-032-30592-3_6

Why Cognitive Assessment in Children Is Important

Relevance to GUIDE

Children's cognitive development strongly influences later educational achievement, career success, psychological wellbeing, and long-term health (Deary et al., 2000; Ritchie & Tucker-Drob, 2018). Similarly, self-regulation and cognitive control, which develop in part in early childhood, are important predictors of long-term success, including better physical health, financial stability, and wellbeing (Moffitt et al., 2013).

Assessing cognitive abilities in childhood is crucial for understanding their development, but also for predicting educational outcomes and ensuring adequate support. A meta-analysis by Roth et al. (2015) found a strong correlation ($\rho = 0.54$) between intelligence and school achievement. Given this connection, assessing cognitive abilities in childhood is essential for understanding developmental trajectories and identifying predictors of later educational and life outcomes, which is why GUIDE includes cognitive measures. While cognitive abilities strongly influence educational achievement, research also suggests a bidirectional relationship between the two. A meta-analysis by Ritchie and Tucker-Drob (2018) indicated that more years spent in education can improve cognitive abilities, suggesting that cognitive development is not fixed but can be shaped by learning. Research by Peng and Kievit (2020) highlights a bidirectional relationship between cognitive abilities and educational outcomes, with better cognitive abilities leading to better academic success and quality education further improving cognitive skills. These research results indicate that cognitive abilities are not static, but dynamic and subject to influences. For this reason, measuring cognitive abilities is crucial for understanding developmental differences across children and for examining how early abilities predict later outcomes, which underpins the rationale for including cognitive measures in GUIDE.

Recognizing the importance of measuring cognitive ability, GUIDE integrates cognitive assessments as a key element of its research design. GUIDE's longitudinal design allows for the investigation of how cognitive abilities develop and how they interact with environmental, social, and educational factors over time. A key reason for introducing cognitive assessments into longitudinal research is their potential to provide insight into patterns of cognitive development and individual differences, including developmental delays and giftedness (Flanagan & Harrison, 2012). Studies such as Growing Up in Ireland (GUI) have shown that assessments of academic skills, attention, and executive function can have the potential to predict later academic achievement and socio-emotional outcomes, highlighting the value of including cognitive measures in longitudinal cohort studies (Williams et al., 2009). This is also a central aim of GUIDE, to explore how early cognitive abilities relate to later educational, social, and wellbeing outcomes (see Chap. 1 in this book). Similarly, the British Cohort Study (BCS70) highlighted the importance of early verbal and nonverbal reasoning tests in predicting career success and higher education

(Elliott & Shepherd, 2006). These findings highlight the role of cognitive assessments within GUIDE as research tools for understanding developmental trajectories and identifying risk and protective factors at the population level. Also, research shows that the impact of early cognitive abilities on later cognitive outcomes is often mediated by the availability of educational resources and socioeconomic conditions in childhood (McElroy et al., 2021). GUIDE offers a unique opportunity to examine these mechanisms further across diverse national contexts with differing educational systems and social policies.

Importance of Cognitive Assessment in Longitudinal Research

Longitudinal designs enable researchers to track developmental trajectories and patterns over time, rather than just assessing current levels of cognitive ability. Cognitive ability measured longitudinally provides evidence supporting potential causal relationships between early abilities and later life outcomes (Casey et al., 2005; Ritchie & Tucker-Drob, 2018). Sensitive periods in cognitive development highlight when population-level interventions, such as early childhood education programs and parenting support, may yield the greatest long-term benefits by capitalizing on brain plasticity during early childhood. Biological factors, including genetic predispositions and prenatal influences, interact with environmental and contextual factors, such as family support and educational resources, to shape cognitive development and later outcomes (see Chap. 7 in this book; Casey et al., 2005). By integrating these perspectives, GUIDE will be able to explore how biological and environmental factors jointly shape cognitive development across different national contexts and over time.

Building on this rationale, the Early Childhood Longitudinal Study (ECLS-K) in the United States showed that early cognitive abilities at school entry related to executive functions such as working memory and cognitive flexibility can predict reading comprehension, success in mathematics, and overall academic success in both elementary and middle school (Morgan et al., 2019; Tourangeau et al., 2015). Within the UK, the Avon Longitudinal Study of Parents and Children (ALSPAC) showed that early cognitive abilities are associated with socio-emotional wellbeing and mental health throughout life (Sullivan et al., 2014). These findings indicate that longitudinal assessment of cognitive abilities can shed light not only on educational outcomes but also on broader aspects of development, including emotional adjustment and mental health. Examining such links helps researchers better understand how cognition and wellbeing evolve together over time, which is also an important aim of GUIDE.

Lessons Learned from Previous Longitudinal Studies

Previous and ongoing large-scale longitudinal studies provide important implications for the development of the cognitive measure in GUIDE. For example, the Early Childhood Longitudinal Study (ECLS) in the United States has shown that combining cognitive, socio-emotional, and contextual data on children leads to a better understanding of child development (Najarian et al., 2020). The ECLS-K project used a wide range of cognitive measures, such as assessments of early literacy, mathematics, and science. They also used teacher and parent assessments of socio-emotional skills and classroom behavior. The combined measures provide an overall holistic perspective and insights into how cognitive abilities and characteristics of the child's environment interact to shape developmental outcomes (Najarian et al., 2020). For GUIDE, this underlines the importance of integrating cognitive data with socio-emotional and contextual measures.

The Dunedin Multidisciplinary Health and Development Study (DMHDS) is a longitudinal study that investigated how children's early cognitive abilities influence later life outcomes (Poulton et al., 2015). It included both verbal and nonverbal tests of children's intelligence and used measures of executive function and specific academic skills such as reading and math. Findings demonstrated that children with low scores on tests of verbal intelligence and executive functions showed a greater tendency to develop later antisocial behavior (Moffitt & Caspi, 2001). For GUIDE, such evidence illustrates how early cognitive assessments can help identify developmental risk factors. The Dunedin study highlights how critical early cognitive assessments are to understand long-term life outcomes. These findings suggest that GUIDE could benefit from including measures of cognitive ability and socio-behavioral outcomes to capture long-term developmental patterns.

The Millennium Cohort Study (MCS) followed approximately 19,000 children born between 2000 and 2002 in the UK, making it one of the largest longitudinal studies. Over the years, they collected data on various aspects of child development. They measured children's cognitive functions, assessments of reading and math skills, executive functions, and attention during childhood and adolescence, as well as assessments of family environment and socioeconomic status (Joshi & Fitzsimons, 2016). The study's findings showed that early cognitive abilities had an impact not only on later school success, but also on socioeconomic status in adulthood (Hansen et al., 2010). Children with higher scores on early cognitive ability tests were more likely to complete higher levels of education and achieve better socioeconomic status. The study also highlights the key role of socioeconomic factors, such as the quality of the family environment and the availability of educational resources, in moderating the effect of cognitive abilities on long-term outcomes (Joshi & Fitzsimons, 2016). These results indicate the need for early interventions to reduce inequalities among children from different cultures and socioeconomic statuses. For GUIDE, this highlights the value of considering socioeconomic factors when interpreting cognitive outcomes and cross-national differences.

The designs of these studies, as well as the findings of some published studies, have important implications for GUIDE. GUIDE should consider integrating cognitive assessment with the collection of socioeconomic and health data to provide a comprehensive picture of children's development and long-term predictors of life success. By including multiple measures and contextual information, GUIDE can further advance understanding of child development and enable more precise policy interventions tailored to the needs of children. Cognitive abilities can be assessed through various approaches, including verbal and nonverbal measures that differ in their dependence on language and cultural context. As the following sections discuss in more detail, these distinctions are particularly relevant for GUIDE when selecting appropriate instruments for use across countries (see Chap. 5 in this book). By using instruments that minimize language barriers, the project ensures fair assessments of cognitive ability and valid cross-national comparisons (see Chap. 9 in this book).

Theoretical Framework of Child Cognitive Development

The study of cognitive abilities and intelligence has been ongoing within the field of psychology for over a century. This section introduces several key theories that have shaped how cognitive abilities are understood and measured, including Spearman's concept of general intelligence, Guilford's multidimensional model, and Cattell's distinction between fluid and crystallized abilities. These approaches were selected because they continue to provide a foundation for understanding individual differences and children's cognitive development.

Cognitive abilities are generally defined as the skills needed to acquire and use knowledge, solve problems, and adapt to new challenges. One of the earliest and most important approaches to measuring cognitive abilities comes from Charles Spearman, who introduced the concept of the *g factor*, or general intelligence, in the early twentieth century. His research showed that people who were successful on certain cognitive tests, such as those measuring verbal, spatial, and numerical abilities, were often good at others, suggesting the presence of a common underlying ability (Spearman, 1961). This general intelligence is closely related to the idea of general cognitive ability, which reflects a person's ability to reason, problem-solve, and learn—abilities that are key to understanding cognitive development.

J. P. Guilford's Structure of Intellect (SI) model introduced a multi-dimensional perspective on cognitive abilities, proposing that intelligence consists of numerous distinct factors rather than a single general ability. His model identified over 100 intellectual abilities categorized into three dimensions: operations (e.g., evaluation, divergent production), contents (e.g., visual, semantic), and products (e.g., units, systems; Guilford, 1967). However, despite its conceptual influence, the model received limited empirical support and was later refined and integrated into a more comprehensive framework.

Raymond Cattell's theory, often referred to as the theory of fluid and crystallized intelligence, highlights an important distinction between these two forms of cognitive ability. Fluid abilities help individuals solve new problems and use abstract reasoning, even when they have no prior knowledge in a field, while crystallized abilities rely on accumulated knowledge and experience throughout life. Research shows that fluid abilities typically peak during early adulthood and then decline with age, while crystallized abilities continue to grow over time, thanks to experience and learning (Cattell, 1963). This distinction is particularly relevant for assessing children's cognitive abilities, as different cognitive skills may mature at different stages.

Children's cognitive development is not linear, but rather a dynamic process with clear changes throughout childhood and adolescence. Early childhood is characterized by rapid development in basic cognitive skills such as memory and attention. As children grow into adolescence, more complex abilities such as abstract thinking and executive functioning become increasingly prominent (Anderson, 2002; Best & Miller, 2010; Horn & Cattell, 1967). Both genetic and environmental factors shape children's cognitive development. Studies show that genes play a significant role, with estimates suggesting that genetic factors account for 50% to 80% of differences in cognitive ability (Plomin & Deary, 2015). However, environmental factors are also important; research highlights the dynamic interplay between genes and environments (Tucker-Drob & Bates, 2016). Parental support, access to education, and socioeconomic status can both help and hinder a child's cognitive development (Bradley & Corwyn, 2002). Longitudinal studies, including GUIDE, highlight how providing a stimulating environment can help children reach their cognitive potential.

Drawing on these theoretical frameworks, GUIDE focuses on assessing general cognitive ability through a single measure. This approach aligns with the longstanding evidence, beginning with Spearman's concept of general intelligence, that performance across different cognitive tasks reflects a common underlying factor. At the same time, using a nonverbal measure allows GUIDE to minimize the influence of language and cultural background, ensuring fair and valid assessment across diverse populations and providing insight into children's developmental potential.

Types of Cognitive Assessments for Children

There are several types of cognitive tests for adults and children. Assessments are categorized by the type of task used to measure cognitive abilities, the mode of administration, and the type of cognitive ability measured. The key distinction is between verbal and nonverbal tests (Flanagan & Harrison, 2012), which are the focus of the next section.

Verbal and Nonverbal Tests

Verbally administered tests of cognitive ability require language skills to understand instructions and respond to the tasks themselves. Individuals who are verbally fluent and have a good understanding of the test language are therefore at an advantage (Sattler, 2008). These tests include tasks such as word definition, sentence completion, and analogies comprehension. The most well-known verbal test is the Wechsler Verbal Comprehension Index, part of the Wechsler Intelligence Scale for Children (WISC). This test assesses a child's ability to understand and produce language (Wechsler, 2014). The Stanford-Binet Intelligence Scale (Roid, 2003) and the Kaufman Assessment Battery for Children (KABC; Kaufman & Kaufman, 1983) are also commonly used in work with children, assessing a range of language-based cognitive skills (Roid, 2003). Verbal cognitive tests are usually administered individually by a trained examiner, often a licensed psychologist, allowing the instructions and testing process to be adapted to the child's needs (Sattler, 2008). This also allows the test administrator to observe nonverbal cues, such as signs of anxiety, fatigue, or difficulty maintaining attention (Kaufman & Lichtenberger, 2005).

Nonverbal cognitive ability tests are used to assess cognitive processes such as abstract reasoning, visuospatial processing, and problem-solving (Wasserman, 2017). These tests do not involve verbal instructions or responses, meaning they are valuable for assessing children with language impairments and those from diverse cultural and linguistic backgrounds, including non-native speakers (Raven, 2000). For example, Raven's Progressive Matrices assess pattern recognition and logical reasoning using visual stimuli (Raven, 2000), while the Naglieri Nonverbal Ability Test (NNAT) uses problem-solving tasks involving geometric shapes and patterns (Naglieri, 2003). A key advantage of nonverbal tests is their ability to reduce the influence of language and cultural influences, leading to a fairer assessment of cognitive ability (Rushton et al., 2003). Nonverbal tests generally measure general cognitive ability, often related to general intelligence (g factor), offering valuable insight into a child's cognitive potential (Anunciação et al., 2024). Their brevity, ease of administration, and reduced dependence on language make them particularly well suited for large-scale, cross-national studies such as GUIDE, where ensuring fairness and comparability across diverse linguistic and cultural contexts is essential.

Individual and Group Tests

Individual tests are administered with one child in a room, with a psychologist as the test administrator. This method of administering the test allows for the adaptation of the test to the child, which includes adjusting the pace and instructions. This type of test is particularly useful for children with learning disabilities or other specific cognitive difficulties. An example of an individual test is the Wechsler Intelligence

Scale for Children (WISC), administered by a psychologist that may adjust the test instructions to ensure that the child fully understands the tasks.

Group tests, commonly administered in educational or research settings, allow efficient data collection assessing cognitive abilities in large numbers of children at once (Demetriou et al., 2020). Although less individualized than one-on-one assessments, group cognitive tests offer several advantages: they can measure abilities in a large number of children in a short period of time, and their use of standardized administration procedures ensures consistent assessment results. This type of testing is more commonly used for nonverbal tests, such as Raven's Progressive Matrices or Naglieri Nonverbal Ability Test (NNAT), as they often rely on visual problem-solving tasks that can be administered equally well in groups (Naglieri, 2003; Raven, 2000). In large-scale studies such as GUIDE, group-administered nonverbal tests provide a practical and fair solution for assessing cognitive abilities across diverse populations.

Tests that Measure General Cognitive Ability and Specific Dimensions

Tests that measure general cognitive ability are designed to assess overall intellectual ability, typically represented by a single score that reflects the g factor. These tests provide an estimate of a child's cognitive potential. Examples of such assessments include Raven's Progressive Matrices and the Naglieri Nonverbal Ability Test (NNAT), which both assess abstract reasoning and general cognitive ability through visual tasks.

Tests that measure specific dimensions of cognitive functioning focus on discrete abilities such as memory, attention, or spatial reasoning, rather than general intelligence. These tests are valuable for diagnosing specific learning disabilities. Examples include subtests from the Wechsler Intelligence Scale for Children (Wechsler, 2014) that assess working memory, processing speed, and verbal comprehension. Additionally, working memory scales are commonly used in educational and clinical settings to assess a child's abilities to retain and manipulate information over short periods, which is critical for tasks involving learning and comprehension (Flanagan & Harrison, 2012). For studies such as GUIDE, the focus on general cognitive ability is particularly valuable because it provides a reliable and comparable indicator of children's overall cognitive functioning across diverse cultural and linguistic contexts.

Considerations in Measuring Cognitive Abilities in Children

When assessing children's cognitive abilities, several key considerations must be considered to ensure valid, fair, and ethical testing. A fundamental consideration of assessing children's cognitive abilities is ensuring that tests are developmentally appropriate and account for differences across ages. Thus, tasks that are interesting, colorful, and interactive, such as simple problem-solving, object manipulation, or picture-based assessments, may be more appropriate for younger children (Hughes & Ensor, 2007), as they help sustain attention and keep children engaged during testing. As children grow older, the complexity of the tasks increases; for example, tasks increasingly involve abstract thinking and verbal problem-solving. Ensuring that the content of the test is consistent with the child's developmental stage is crucial for obtaining accurate and meaningful results of cognitive assessment of children (Anderson, 2001; Best & Miller, 2010).

Another consideration when measuring children's cognitive abilities is cultural sensitivity. Cultural norms and values significantly influence how children approach problem-solving and understand the tasks in the test itself (Helms-Lorenz et al., 2003). Tests that rely on specific cultural knowledge, such as verbal analogies, may disadvantage children from different linguistic or cultural backgrounds. Culturally sensitive tests, such as Raven's Progressive Matrices or the Naglieri Nonverbal Ability Test, minimize reliance on language and culturally biased content by focusing on universal cognitive processes such as pattern recognition (Rushton et al., 2003). This approach ensures that children from different cultural contexts are assessed fairly, thereby reducing the risk of language bias (Van de Vijver & Tanzer, 2004).

In testing children's cognitive abilities, it is important to ensure a fair and ethical approach in assessment (see Chap. 2 in this book). Fairness involves minimizing biases related to language, culture, gender, or socioeconomic status, which is also essential for ensuring the reliability and validity of test results (Suzuki & Ponterotto, 2007). Those administering the test must ensure consistency in the testing conditions. All children should understand the instructions before testing begins (Gregory, 2004). Ethical considerations include obtaining informed consent from parents or caregivers, obtaining informed assent from children themselves, and ensuring that test results are used appropriately in accordance with the principles of psychological testing (American Psychological Association, 2017; Matarazzo, 1990). These ethical guidelines are essential for maintaining the integrity of the assessment process and protecting the child's wellbeing (American Psychological Association, 2017).

Evaluation of Nonverbal Cognitive Assessment in GUIDE

The main advantage of using a nonverbal cognitive test in GUIDE is that it allows for a fair assessment of the cognitive abilities of children from diverse linguistic and regional backgrounds. This is crucial in the longitudinal design of GUIDE, as it allows for valid comparisons across countries and populations, ensuring that the results reflect cognitive abilities rather than cultural or linguistic differences. Additionally, the administration of nonverbal tests is highly standardized, reducing variability in test conditions and ensuring reliability across different settings and overtime, which makes them particularly suitable for longitudinal studies such as GUIDE. Unlike many traditional cognitive assessments that require a trained psychologist, the nonverbal test planned for use in GUIDE will be administered by trained survey interviewers, allowing for large-scale implementation while maintaining consistency in data collection. GUIDE's nonverbal test of general cognitive ability will allow fair comparison of children's performances across different languages and cultures and track their cognitive development over time.

Administration of Cognitive Assessment and Interpretation of Results

Cognitive ability testing with children involves following standardized testing procedures to ensure reliability and validity (Embretson & Reise, 2013). Test administrators must be thoroughly trained in the administration of the test itself, with the aim of reducing examiner effects. Training should also include familiarity with the test instructions (including how to deliver instructions consistently and convey them to children without compromising the standardization of test administration), manage unexpected child behavior, and maintain controlled testing conditions that minimize distractions (Jafari et al., 2019). Establishing a calm and supportive atmosphere helps reduce anxiety and yields more accurate results (Flanagan & Harrison, 2012). Simple techniques, such as explaining the purpose of the test in child-friendly language and starting with easy tasks, can help children feel at ease. In GUIDE, standardized testing protocols across countries are essential for collecting comparable and reliable data.

Test results must be interpreted in the context of developmental norms and individual differences. Developmental norms represent the average scores of a population of children of the same age and are used to assess whether a child's performance is within expected developmental limits. By comparing performance with age-appropriate reference values, it is possible to identify areas of strength as well as potential developmental difficulties (Wechsler, 2014). When interpreting results, it is important to consider the broader context, including socioeconomic background, availability of educational resources, and parental involvement. Children who grew up in different environments may not have had equal opportunities to develop certain skills, so test results need to be interpreted in context to avoid confusing environmental disadvantage with lower ability and to ensure valid cross-country comparisons. For example, a child from a family with fewer educational resources may perform lower on verbal tasks, but this may not reflect their actual intelligence, but rather the circumstances in which they grew up (Hart & Risley, 2003). Building on these considerations, GUIDE goes a step further than simply assessing scores. By integrating cognitive scores with information about socioeconomic status, school environment, and family circumstances, it provides a holistic view of each child's development. This approach helps distinguish situations where a child is truly struggling from those where challenges are the result of external circumstances. This evidence can inform educational and social policies aimed at promoting equitable developmental opportunities for all children.

Ethical Issues in Testing Children's Cognitive Abilities

In testing with children, it is necessary to request and obtain informed consent to participate in the research from the child's parents or caregivers (see Chaps. 2 and 3 in this book). Informed consent must include an explanation of the purpose of the testing, what will be measured by the research, and an explanation of how the results will be used (American Psychological Association, 2017; Morrow & Richards, 1996). Also, before conducting the test, it is necessary to inform the children themselves about the purpose of the research.

Test results must be treated as sensitive data and stored in a secure manner to protect the child's privacy (see Chap. 8 in this book). In research contexts such as GUIDE, access to identifiable information is strictly limited to authorized research personnel. To protect participants' privacy while allowing data linkage across waves and informants, all data are pseudonymized and stored securely in accordance with data protection regulations (American Psychological Association, 2017). GUIDE follows international ethical guidelines, with protocols in place to protect the privacy and wellbeing of participants. Particular attention is paid to vulnerable populations, ensuring that assessments do not reinforce inequalities or lead to labeling.

Conclusion and Recommendations

Cognitive assessment is essential for understanding patterns of child development and the factors that influence them. Within GUIDE, the selection of a single, nonverbal measure of general cognitive ability ensures a fair, inclusive, and comparable assessment that is independent of the child's language or cultural background. By using a nonverbal test that focuses on the general intelligence factor (g factor), GUIDE can provide valuable data on children's cognitive development in different settings across Europe.

Large studies, such as the Dunedin Interdisciplinary Study of Health and Development and the Millennium Cohort Study, demonstrate the value of integrating cognitive data with broader developmental information. This approach helps identify additional factors influencing children's development and can inform educational and social policies aimed at reducing inequalities and promoting equal opportunities. GUIDE embraces this holistic approach from other longitudinal studies linking cognitive data with information on children's social and educational backgrounds. This integration is crucial for identifying key factors influencing children's development, enabling researchers to inform effective educational and social policies aimed at reducing inequalities and promoting equal opportunities for children across Europe.

References

American Psychological Association. (2017). *Ethical principles of psychologists and code of conduct*. https://www.apa.org/ethics/code/

Anderson, P. (2002). Assessment and development of executive function (EF) during childhood. *Child Neuropsychology, 8*(2), 71–82. https://doi.org/10.1076/chin.8.2.71.8724

Anderson, V. (2001). Assessing executive functions in children: Biological, psychological, and developmental considerations. *Pediatric Rehabilitation, 4*(3), 119–136. https://doi.org/10.1080/13638490110091347

Anunciação, L., Marques, L., Murray, C., Portugal, A. C., Rabelo, I., Landeira-Fernandez, J., & Cruz, R. (2024). Psychometric properties of a brief non-verbal test of *g* factor intelligence. *Journal of Psychological Perspectives, 6*(1), 47–62.

Best, J. R., & Miller, P. H. (2010). A developmental perspective on executive function. *Child Development, 81*(6), 1641–1660. https://doi.org/10.1111/j.1467-8624.2010.01499.x

Bradley, R. H., & Corwyn, R. F. (2002). Socioeconomic status and child development. *Annual Review of Psychology, 53*, 371–399. https://doi.org/10.1146/annurev.psych.53.100901.135233

Casey, B. J., Tottenham, N., Liston, C., & Durston, S. (2005). Imaging the developing brain: What have we learned about cognitive development? *Trends in Cognitive Sciences, 9*(3), 104–110. https://doi.org/10.1016/j.tics.2005.01.011

Cattell, R. B. (1963). Theory of fluid and crystallized intelligence: A critical experiment. *Journal of Educational Psychology, 54*(1), 1–22. https://doi.org/10.1037/h0046743

Demetriou, A., Kazi, S., Makris, N., & Spanoudis, G. (2020). Cognitive ability, cognitive self-awareness, and school performance: From childhood to adolescence. *Intelligence, 79*, Article 101432. https://doi.org/10.1016/j.intell.2020.101432

Deary, I. J., Whalley, L. J., Lemmon, H., Crawford, J. R., & Starr, J. M. (2000). The stability of individual differences in mental ability from childhood to old age: Follow-up of the 1932 Scottish Mental Survey. *Intelligence, 28*(1), 49–55. https://doi.org/10.1016/S0160-2896(99)00031-8

Elliott, J., & Shepherd, P. (2006). Cohort profile: 1970 British Birth Cohort (BCS70). *International Journal of Epidemiology, 35*(4), 836–843. https://doi.org/10.1093/ije/dyl174

Embretson, S. E., & Reise, S. P. (2013). *Item response theory for psychologists*. Psychology Press.

Flanagan, D. P., & Harrison, P. L. (Eds.). (2012). *Contemporary intellectual assessment: Theories, tests, and issues* (3rd ed.). Guilford Press.

Gregory, R. J. (2004). *Psychological testing: History, principles, and applications* (4th ed.). Pearson Education India.

Guilford, J. P. (1967). *The nature of human intelligence*. McGraw-Hill.

Hansen, K., Jones, E., Joshi, H., & Budge, D. (2010). *Millennium Cohort Study fourth survey: A user's guide to initial findings*. Centre for Longitudinal Studies. https://cls.ucl.ac.uk/wp-content/uploads/2017/07/MCS4-Users-Guide-to-Initial-Findings-2nd-Edition-15-12-10_MT.pdf

Hart, B., & Risley, T. R. (2003). The early catastrophe: The 30 million word gap by age 3. *American Educator, 27*(1), 4–9.

Helms-Lorenz, M., Van de Vijver, F. J. R., & Poortinga, Y. H. (2003). Cross-cultural differences in cognitive performance and Spearman's hypothesis: *G* or *c*? *Intelligence, 31*(1), 9–29. https://doi.org/10.1016/S0160-2896(02)00111-3

Horn, J. L., & Cattell, R. B. (1967). Age differences in fluid and crystallized intelligence. *Acta Psychologica, 26*(2), 107–129. https://doi.org/10.1016/0001-6918(67)90011-X

Hughes, C., & Ensor, R. (2007). Executive function and theory of mind: Predictive relations from ages 2 to 4. *Developmental Psychology, 43*(6), 1447–1459. https://doi.org/10.1037/0012-1649.43.6.1447

Jafari, M. J., Khosrowabadi, R., Khodakarim, S., & Mohammadian, F. (2019). The effect of noise exposure on cognitive performance and brain activity patterns. *Open Access Macedonian Journal of Medical Sciences, 7*(17), 2924–2931. https://doi.org/10.3889/oamjms.2019.742

Joshi, H., & Fitzsimons, E. (2016). The Millennium Cohort Study: The making of a multi-purpose resource for social science and policy. *Longitudinal and Life Course Studies, 7*(4), 409–430. https://doi.org/10.14301/llcs.v7i4.410

Kaufman, A. S., & Kaufman, N. L. (1983). *Kaufman assessment battery for children*. American Guidance Service.

Kaufman, A. S., & Lichtenberger, E. O. (2005). *Assessing adolescent and adult intelligence* (3rd ed.). John Wiley & Sons.

Matarazzo, J. D. (1990). Psychological assessment versus psychological testing: Validation from Binet to the school, clinic, and courtroom. *American Psychologist, 45*(9), 999–1017. https://doi.org/10.1037/0003-066X.45.9.999

McElroy, E., Richards, M., Fitzsimons, E., Conti, G., Ploubidis, G. B., Sullivan, A., & Moulton, V. (2021). Influence of childhood socioeconomic position and ability on mid-life cognitive function: Evidence from three British birth cohorts. *Journal of Epidemiology and Community Health, 75*(7), 643–650. https://doi.org/10.1136/jech-2020-215637

Moffitt, T. E., & Caspi, A. (2001). Childhood predictors differentiate life-course-persistent and adolescence-limited antisocial pathways among males and females. *Development and Psychopathology, 13*(2), 355–375. https://doi.org/10.1017/S0954579401002097

Moffitt, T. E., Poulton, R., & Caspi, A. (2013). Lifelong impact of early self-control. *American Scientist, 101*(5), 352–359. https://doi.org/10.1511/2013.104.352

Morgan, P. L., Farkas, G., Wang, Y., Hillemeier, M. M., Oh, Y., & Maczuga, S. (2019). Executive function deficits in kindergarten predict repeated academic difficulties across elementary school. *Early Childhood Research Quarterly, 46*, 20–32. https://doi.org/10.1016/j.ecresq.2018.06.009

Morrow, V., & Richards, M. (1996). The ethics of social research with children: An overview. *Children & Society, 10*(2), 90–105. https://doi.org/10.1111/j.1099-0860.1996.tb00461.x

Naglieri, J. A. (2003). Naglieri nonverbal ability tests: NNAT and MAT-EF. In R. S. McCallum (Ed.), *Handbook of nonverbal assessment* (pp. 175–189). Springer.

Najarian, M., Tourangeau, K., Nord, C., Wallner-Allen, K., Vaden-Kiernan, N., & Mulligan, G. M. (2020). *Early Childhood Longitudinal Study, Kindergarten Class of 2010–11 (ECLS-K:2011): User's manual for the kindergarten-fifth grade data file and electronic codebook, public version* (NCES 2020-123). National Center for Education Statistics.

Peng, P., & Kievit, R. A. (2020). The development of academic achievement and cognitive abilities: A bidirectional perspective. *Child Development Perspectives, 14*(1), 15–20. https://doi.org/10.1111/cdep.12352

Plomin, R., & Deary, I. J. (2015). Genetics and intelligence differences: Five special findings. *Molecular Psychiatry, 20*(1), 98–108. https://doi.org/10.1038/mp.2014.105

Poulton, R., Moffitt, T. E., & Silva, P. A. (2015). The Dunedin multidisciplinary health and development study: Overview of the first 40 years, with an eye to the future. *Social Psychiatry and Psychiatric Epidemiology, 50*(5), 679–693. https://doi.org/10.1007/s00127-015-1048-8

Raven, J. (2000). The Raven's progressive matrices: Change and stability over culture and time. *Cognitive Psychology, 41*(1), 1–48. https://doi.org/10.1006/cogp.1999.0735

Roid, G. H. (2003). *Stanford-Binet Intelligence Scales* (5th ed.). Riverside Publishing.

Roth, B., Becker, N., Romeyke, S., Schäfer, S., Domnick, F., & Spinath, F. M. (2015). Intelligence and school grades: A meta-analysis. *Intelligence, 53*, 118–137. https://doi.org/10.1016/j.intell.2015.09.002

Ritchie, S. J., & Tucker-Drob, E. M. (2018). How much does education improve intelligence? A meta-analysis. *Psychological Science, 29*(8), 1358–1369. https://doi.org/10.1177/0956797618774253

Rushton, J. P., Skuy, M., & Fridjhon, P. (2003). Performance on Raven's advanced progressive matrices by African, East Indian, and White engineering students in South Africa. *Intelligence, 31*(2), 123–137. https://doi.org/10.1016/S0160-2896(02)00140-X

Sattler, J. M. (2008). *Assessment of children: Cognitive foundations* (5th ed.). J. M. Sattler.

Spearman, C. (1961). "General intelligence" objectively determined and measured. In J. J. Jenkins & D. G. Paterson (Eds.), *Studies in individual differences: The search for intelligence* (pp. 59–73). Appleton-Century-Crofts. https://doi.org/10.1037/11491-006

Sternberg, R. J. (2021). *Adaptive intelligence: Surviving and thriving in times of uncertainty.* Cambridge University Press.

Sullivan, S. A., Wiles, N., Kounali, D., Lewis, G., Heron, J., Cannon, M., Mahedy, L., Jones, P. B., Stochl, J., & Zammit, S. (2014). Longitudinal associations between adolescent psychotic experiences and depressive symptoms. *PLOS ONE, 9*(8), Article e105758. https://doi.org/10.1371/journal.pone.0105758

Suzuki, L. A., & Ponterotto, J. G. (Eds.). (2007). *Handbook of multicultural assessment: Clinical, psychological, and educational applications* (3rd ed.). John Wiley & Sons.

Tourangeau, K., Nord, C., Lê, T., Sorongon, A. G., Hagedorn, M. C., Daly, P., & Najarian, M. (2015). *Early Childhood Longitudinal Study, Kindergarten Class of 2010–11 (ECLS-K:2011): User's manual for the ECLS-K:2011 kindergarten data file and electronic codebook, public version* (NCES 2015-074). National Center for Education Statistics. https://nces.ed.gov/pubs2015/2015074.pdf

Tucker-Drob, E. M., & Bates, T. C. (2016). Large cross-national differences in gene × socioeconomic status interaction on intelligence. *Psychological Science, 27*(2), 138–149. https://doi.org/10.1177/0956797615612727

Van de Vijver, F. J. R., & Tanzer, N. K. (2004). Bias and equivalence in cross-cultural assessment: An overview. *European Review of Applied Psychology, 54*(2), 119–135. https://doi.org/10.1016/j.erap.2003.12.004

Wasserman, J. D. (2017). Nonverbal neuropsychological assessment. In R. S. McCallum (Ed.), *Handbook of nonverbal assessment* (2nd ed., pp. 287–310). Springer International Publishing.

Wechsler, D. (2014). *Wechsler intelligence scale for children* (5th ed.). Pearson.

Williams, J., Greene, S., Doyle, E., Harris, E., Layte, R., McCoy, S., McCrory, C., Murray, A., Nixon, E., O'Dowd, T., O'Moore, M., Quail, A., Smyth, E., Swords, L., & Thornton, M. (2009). *Growing up in Ireland: The national longitudinal study of children—The lives of 9-year-olds* (Child Cohort Research Report No. 1). The Stationery Office. https://www.growingup.gov.ie/pubs/BKMNEXT154.pdf

Iva Černja Rajter (Ph.D.) is a postdoc at the Institute of Social Sciences Ivo Pilar and an assistant professor at the University of Zagreb. She earned her Ph.D. in 2022, specializes in career development, and is involved in several research projects, including Horizon Europe research project Growing Up in Digital Europe Preparation Phase (GUIDEPREP).

Toni Babarović (Ph.D.) is a professor at the Department of Psychology, University of Split, Croatia. His research focuses on educational psychology, particularly in areas such as career decision-making, school effectiveness, and educational management. He has contributed to various publications, including studies on career decision-making difficulties and the role of parents' beliefs in students' motivation and achievement.

Ivan Dević (Ph.D.) has been a senior research associate at the Institute of Social Sciences Ivo Pilar since 2009. His research focuses on the wellbeing of children and adults, educational psychology, and career choice. Actively engaged in academic teaching, scientific research, and publishing. He has authored over 25 scientific papers and presented at over 50 conferences.

Chapter 7
Beyond Self-Report: Possibilities and Considerations for Biological Data Collection with Children Across Contexts

Candace Currie and Juliet McEachran

Purpose of the Biological Indicators and Social Research Chapter

Specific objectives of this chapter are:

- To outline the biological indicators to be considered and their sampling.
- To provide a framework for the selection of biological indicators.
- To suggest biological indicators to be included in GUIDE.

Biological Indicators and GUIDE

GUIDE will track the development, wellbeing, and health of children, adolescents, and young adults in the first two and a half decades of their lives in multiple European countries. To understand child development and health over time, and compare these across countries, it is crucial to include biological as well as psychological, social, cultural, economic, and environmental determinants, dimensions, and outcomes. This chapter presents an overview of best practice on the collection and use of child and adolescent biological indicators from relevant scientific literature, published work on existing relevant cohort studies worldwide, and insights shared in discussion with key experts in the field of biological indicators of child and adolescent health. These experts are listed in Appendix A.

C. Currie (✉)
University College London, London, UK
e-mail: candace.currie@ucl.ac.uk

J. McEachran
Glasgow Caledonian University, London, UK

L. K. Taylor et al. (eds.), *Growing Up in Digital Europe*, Springer Series on Child and Family Studies, https://doi.org/10.1007/978-3-032-30592-3_7

Box 7.1 Concepts and Definitions in this Chapter

Biological indicator: an umbrella term for biomarkers and biological measures.

Biomarker: a biological molecule found in blood or other biospecimen that is a sign of a normal or abnormal process, condition, or disease. For example, C-reactive protein (inflammation), cortisol (stress), or an epigenetic marker such as methylation.

Biological measures: an assessment or measure of a physiological process, for example height and weight (growth).

Biospecimen: a biological sample. For example, blood or urine.

The bioecological model (see Chap. 1 in this book) provides a conceptual framework to identify relevant biological indicators. This model places the growing and developing child, adolescent, and young adult within their physical, social, and cultural environment, measured at different system levels (Bronfenbrenner & Ceci, 1994; Currie & Morgan, 2020, 2024). Individual factors affecting health and development include growth and pubertal maturation, genetics, socio-demographic characteristics, and behaviors. Environmental factors that affect biological processes in positive and negative ways can be found at the individual, micro-, meso-, and macro-levels within the bioecological framework.

> Biomarkers help us understand the pathways by which the environment gets under the skin. (Benzeval, 2017)

To explore how the environment influences these biological processes in practice, it is useful to unpack the specific determinants found at each level of this framework. At the individual level, a range of behaviors are important to consider as determinants of biological processes underlying health and development. These include dietary habits, physical activity, sleep, social media consumption, the use of nicotine, drugs and alcohol, and health service use. There is a rich literature on a range of micro-level determinants that may positively or negatively affect health, including food insecurity, nurturing social relationships, neglect and abuse, and exposures to harmful environmental substances such as metals, particulate matter, phthalates in plastics, and growth hormones in foods. These various factors can all impact the biological processes of healthy development, including emotional health, physical development, neurodevelopment, and reproductive development. Meso-level factors operate at the community level, including elements such as access to sports facilities and green space, neighborhood violence and drug use, safety, and security. These determinants can affect outcomes such as stress, physical activity, substance use, and being a victim of violence. Macro-level determinants, which are crucial for understanding health and development in different countries, include country-level health profile, wealth and socioeconomic inequalities, and national health, education, and social policies (Currie & Morgan, 2020, 2024).

In the following sections, biological indicators collected by previous cohorts are discussed, as are the sampling methods employed. Specific biospecimens and the biomarkers available in these specimens are examined to provide estimates of the cost of collecting biological indicators. Finally, a suggestion is made about what GUIDE could collect. The selection of biological indicators in longitudinal social surveys is a balance of research priorities, participant burden, ethical considerations (see also Chap. 2 in this book), and cost and allowance for technological and academic advances (see also Chap. 10 in this book) that will be made during the lifespan of the cohort.

Biological Indicators

Since the sequencing of the human genome in 2003, there has been a rapid series of technological advances that now allow social surveys to also collect genomic data at scale, with the Millenium Cohort Study (MCS) and the Longitudinal Study of Australian Children (LSAC) both collecting genetic data for the first time in 2015. Similar advances have been made in the identification of other biomarkers crucial to health and development. GUIDE can capitalize on this knowhow and integrate biological indicators, including genetic and epigenetic biomarkers, into its scope to maximize its potential now and in the future.

Ground-breaking cohorts such as the UK Avon Longitudinal Study of Parents and Children (ALSPAC; Fraser et al., 2013) and the New Zealand Dunedin Study (Poulton et al., 2015) were initiated before the biomarkers era, predating the identification and economic feasibility of including the broad range of biological indicators now available in large population cohorts. This chapter concentrates on recent birth, infant, or adolescent cohorts which have gathered a range of biological indicators and have the following characteristics:

- Focused on infant, child, and adolescent wellbeing and development beyond perinatal epidemiology.
- Data collection began in 2000 or later.
- Collected more than anthropometric data from infants, children, and/or adolescents.
- Had a sample of greater than 500 that was representative of the broader population.

Indicators Collected

The biological indicators collected, and the sampling methods employed by 30 existing cohorts, are summarized throughout this chapter and detailed in Appendix B. Anthropometric measures, for example height and weight, were collected by all but one of the 30 cohorts. The mean number of biological indicators collected by a cohort was 6.1 out of a total of 30. Fifteen surveys collected five or less biological indicators or biospecimens (Table 7.1).

Table 7.1 Biological measures and biospecimens collected by selected cohorts

Biological measures	N
Anthropometrics, including body composition and bone density	29
Blood pressure and heart rate	16
Lung function	7
Pubertal measures	7
Physical activity, including accelerometry and cycle ergometry	8
Skin prick test[a]	3
Grip strength	3
Carotid artery scan	2
Brain imaging[a]	2
Hearing[a]	2
Dental observations	1
Thyroid[a]	1
Menstrual data	1
Biospecimens	
Blood, including venous, peripheral blood, and dried blood	17
Urine	15
Saliva	10
Hair	9
Fecal biome/stool	7
Teeth	6
Buccal swab	4
Nails	3
Nasal swab	1
Breath	1
Environmental indicators	
Mite allergen/endotoxin in house dust	4
Indoor gaseous atmospheric contaminants	3

[a]These measures were collected by few cohorts and require clinic-based equipment and as a result are not further discussed in this chapter. Breast milk, meconium, placenta, umbilical cord tissue, and umbilical cord blood were also collected in some surveys, but for GUIDE the data collection window starts at 8 months.

Sampling of Biological Indicators

The collection of biological indicators can be expensive, with some requiring specialist equipment, medically trained staff, respondents to attend clinics, or respondents to appropriately collect and send in biospecimens. Due to these expenses, previous cohorts have used different sampling strategies to reduce costs.

These strategies often involve reducing the number of participants or time points sampled, and the cohorts reviewed provided several examples of this in practice. The approaches generally fall into four categories: (1) collection at a single time point, observed in (a) the MCS (saliva only; Fitzsimons et al., 2022) and (b) LSAC cohort B (16 different types of biological indicators; Clifford et al., 2019); (2) sampling based on a power calculation, where (a) the Japan Environment and Children's Study (JECS; Michikawa et al., 2015) and (b) the French national cohort of children (ELFE; Charles et al., 2020) sampled only 44% of all maternity units rather than the full population; (3) using subsamples for specific waves while sampling all respondents at others, illustrated by (a) the Generation R Study (GenR; Jaddoe et al., 2006), which used a sub-sample among those under 6 years and sampled all thereafter, and (b) Born in Bradford (BiB; Wright et al., 2013), which conducted specific sub-studies for children under 6 before sampling the full cohort from 6 years onwards; and (4) restricting sampling to original geographic areas, seen in (a) the German Health Interview and Examination Survey for Children and Adolescents (KiGGS; Mauz et al., 2020), which restricted biological sampling to the original primary sampling units at Wave 2 to avoid the cost of setting up clinics nationwide, and (b) the MCS, which similarly benefited from utilizing its original sampling frame of specific local council wards (Fitzsimons et al., 2022).

The location where biological indicators were collected clearly illustrates design choices aimed at facilitating the process. Across the cohorts reviewed, the primary collection sites varied: nine cohorts collected data in the respondent's home, nine utilized a clinic, and six employed a combination of home and clinic visits at different study waves. Fewer cohorts used schools (two) or a combination of homes and schools (one). Additionally, one cohort relied solely on linked records, while the collection location for one other remained unspecified.

At a time when social surveys are moving to be collected online/remotely, the inclusion of some biological indicators can necessitate contact between research staff and respondents and others require respondents to attend a clinic. There are a variety of different sampling models for collecting biological indicators: data collection in clinic, school, or home; 100% sampling; clinical subsampling; targeted age-specific data collection; or collection at each wave of data collection.

These examples highlight that obtaining biological data is rarely a straightforward process, but rather a series of strategic compromises. Depending on who is tested, where data is collected, and how frequently sampling occurs, researchers can successfully gather essential biological evidence while maintaining the study's financial and logistical viability.

Drawing on a review of best practices in scientific literature, an analysis of existing global cohort studies, and insights gained from discussions with key experts in the field (see Expert Consultations in Appendix A), three primary categories of biological indicators regarding the wellbeing of children, adolescents, and young adults have been identified. The following sections detail these domains: Biological Measures (i.e., anthropometric measures, blood pressure and pulse, lung function, and physical activity and fitness), Biospecimens (i.e., saliva, hair, nails, teeth, blood, buccal swabs, urine, and fecal biome/stools), and Other Health Data (i.e., objective and wider health data, linked data, environmental indicators, and linked environmental data). In addition, the pros and cons of different biological indicators in the context of a nationally representative population have been summarized in Table 7.2.

Biological Measures

Anthropometric Measures

Anthropometric measures include height, weight, body composition, circumference (e.g., arm and waist) and skin fold measures (e.g., triceps), many of which are measurable with simple instruments. Height and weight were the most frequently collected biological indicators in the cohorts examined and it can be argued that, for population-based surveys, BMI (measured by weight (kg)/height $(m)^2$) is the most robust and practical indicator of normal weight, overweight, obesity, and underweight for population statistics (referencing expert consultation with Sean Cumming).

BMI for age charts produced by the World Health Organization can be used to determine whether measurements fall in normal, underweight, overweight, or obese ranges (https://www.who.int/tools/child-growth-standards). Underweight and overweight are both potentially harmful to health and wellbeing from childhood through adulthood (Jebeile et al., 2022). As well as a risk factor for metabolic disease, obesity has been identified as a determining factor in earlier onset of puberty, which is itself a risk factor for a variety of short- and longer-term health problems. For example, being overweight during adolescence is associated with depression, especially among girls. A recent review found that across Europe the prevalence of underweight is considerable (overall, around 8–9%), particularly in Eastern Europe, and follows a slight upward trend during the past decade (Garrido-Miguel et al., 2021). The relationship between psychosocial health and body mass index (BMI) among adolescents in five European countries found that poorer psychosocial health is associated with both under and overweight deviations from normal weight (Drosopoulou et al., 2021). Height measured annually can also be used to assess stages of pubertal development from peak height velocity (Cole, 2018; Granados et al., 2015).

Blood Pressure and Pulse

Blood pressure and pulse (to measure heart rate) can be collected either in a clinic or by a trained interviewer using simple non-invasive instruments. These measurements are affected by time of day as well as stress and exercise. Standardized reading can indicate whether the young person's measurements are within normal or clinical ranges and whether these indicate overall health as well as underlying health issues.

Table 7.2 Pros and cons of collecting different biological indicators in a birth cohort

Biological indicators	Pros	Cons	Biomarkers
Height & weight	Routine, familiar Collected at home	–	BMI
Wearable devices	Data collected independent of research team	–	BP, Physical activity
Saliva	Minimally invasive	Could be difficult to ensure no food or drink for 60 min before saliva is collected Prone to contamination	CRP IL-1β Cortisol
Hair	Minimally invasive Sample at home and post Stored at room temperature Can be collected at any time of day	Cultural and religious sensitivities to collection of hair, especially if head coverings used Reluctance as large sample required Time it takes to regrow hair	Previous months HPA activity, Heavy metals, Drugs
Nails	Minimally invasive Sample at home and post Stored at room temperature	Expensive to process It is difficult to identify exact timing of exposure	Heavy metals, Alcohol and Other Drugs (AOD) DNA
Primary teeth	Opportunity for participant engagement Not invasive Low-cost visual processing for dental health data Sample at home and post Stored at room temperature	Dependent on the parent sending tooth If a tooth is diseased, the parent may not return it out of shame Expensive processing for pollutants and psychological distress data	Dental health, Heavy metals, Psychological distress, DNA
Full blood	If stored aliquots can be used for future research/future proofs study Source of large range, variety and new biomarkers Likely source of new biomarkers	Invasive, costly to collect (trained medical researcher), transport (refrigerated), and process Some are reluctant to share genetic data	Telomere length, Methylation data, DNA/RNA, Cortisol, Inflammation, AOD

(continued)

Table 7.2 (continued)

Biological indicators	Pros	Cons	Biomarkers
Dried blood spots	Once dry, it can be stored at room temperature More cost-effective option than venous blood Less stressful for infants and children Less volume required	Degradation	DNA/RNA, Cholesterol CRP IL-6
Buccal swab	Minimally invasive, no refrigeration	Low RNA/DNA concentration compared to other sources	IL-1β RNA/DNA
Urine	Some biomarkers are easier to detect in urine compared to blood	Respondent discomfort Refrigerated transport	–
Fecal	Easy to collect from nappies (infants)	This is emerging evidence base, and would have to be stored until knowledge and techniques advance Respondent discomfort with feces	Volume and diversity of microbiome
Linked data	Existing data No participant burden	It can be difficult to access Cost to incorporate	BMI, Eye, Teeth, and others

Note Adapted from (Verhoeven et al., 2024)

Pulse rate is a measure of fitness, part of a more extensive set of indicators. A European initiative has developed reference values for health-related fitness in European children and adolescents aged 6–18 years using multiple measures and providing comparisons across European countries (Ortega et al., 2023).

Lung Function

A spirometer is a relatively cheap instrument to measure lung function, and this more basic testing of lung function can be undertaken in the home or at a clinic. Lung function in children and young people is largely related to asthma and other respiratory conditions, and measurements will indicate whether function is within normal or clinical ranges. Environmental pollution is an important factor in respiratory function in children.

Physical Activity and Fitness

Wearable devices such as a pedometer or accelerometer provide an objective measure of activity. Pedometers measure steps while accelerometers also capture the intensity of activity. The data can also be collected via mobile phones and questionnaires. Physical fitness tests can also be conducted in the field using standardized protocols that have been shown to be indicative of key fitness attributes such as strength, power, agility, endurance, and balance. In a laboratory, VO2 max measures the volume of oxygen absorbed while exercising.

Biospecimens

Saliva

Saliva is fluid produced by the salivary glands in the mouth and is 99% water and 1% protein. There is a positive correlation between some biomarker concentrations in blood and saliva, including cortisol, progesterone, and estrogen (Huang et al., 2023). In longitudinal trials, the salivary bacterial community is of particular interest. Saliva samples represent various ecological habitats in the oral cavity and collection of saliva is a non-invasive procedure and thereby convenient for young children (Davis et al., 2023; Eriksen et al., 2024). There is potential for the oral microbiome in early life (Gomez & Nelson, 2017) and the development of salivary diagnostic tools to predict and prevent future oral and systemic disease by analyzing and altering the infant's oral microbiome. Davis and colleagues (2023) describe saliva as a good medium to measure biomarkers in children because samples can be collected repeatedly in a short amount of time or spaced throughout the day. For example, the measurement of diurnal cortisol requires up to 4 samples per day for at least 2 days. This is possible via saliva samples. Saliva samples do not need to be refrigerated, so they are more straightforward to collect than urine.

It is known that child exposure to stressors can affect their immune function, causing inflammation which in turn can have negative effects on health. A recent study has reviewed appropriate biomarkers to measure both the effects of stress and subsequent inflammatory responses (Davis et al., 2023). Common biomarkers of chronic inflammation in children are C-reactive protein (CRP), TNF-α, and IL-6. Similarly, other biomarkers of inflammation, such as IL-2 and IL-1β, may also be considered. CRP and IL-1β can both be detected in saliva.

Saliva can also be used to assess pubertal development corresponding to increases in salivary testosterone, DHEA, estradiol, and progesterone levels throughout adolescence (Omary et al., 2025). Full details of assaying are provided in this paper.

Hair

The analysis of approximately a centimeter of hair, measured from the scalp, can test long-term HPA (hypothalamus pituitary adrenal) axis activity via cortisol and cortisone levels, and also exposure to narcotics and pollutants in the previous month. The HPA axis is activated in response to acute and chronic stress. When it is repeatedly activated under chronic stress, the cortisol hormone is released by the adrenal gland. As hair provides a measure of the previous month's HPA activity, this makes it the ideal choice for the assessment of stress in a population-level longitudinal cohort study, as the timing of sampling during the day is not important.

Nails

Similarly to hair, nails provide information on exposure to pollutants, but there is a greater time lag between the sample being available and the time of exposure to pollutants. It is also possible to measure cortisol and DNA/RNA information from nails. Toenails provide information on the 7–12 months prior to sampling, and fingernails the previous six months. Nails can be a source of information on exposure to heavy metals, but further work is needed to accurately assess the timing of exposure (Salcedo-Bellido et al., 2021).

Teeth

Primary (baby) teeth are the least invasive biospecimen available from children since they are shed naturally and can be easily collected and stored. They facilitate three different measures pertinent to healthy development: (1) caries (dental health), (2) exposure to heavy metals, and (3) psychological distress in early life. Teeth are especially useful for identifying heavy metal pollution due to the propensity of heavy metals to become part of teeth and bone. This makes teeth preferable to blood as the biospecimen by which to examine heavy metal pollution. Teeth have rings, so that the timing of exposure to heavy metals and distress can be determined. Teeth can also provide an estimate of maturation, but stronger measures—for example, skeletal hand and wrist X-rays—are available.

Blood

Blood samples may be collected via venipuncture, finger prick, or heel stick, and provide a plethora of known biomarkers and others yet to be identified when new technologies are developed. New biomarkers will most likely first be identified in blood; therefore, the collection of blood is a means by which a longitudinal study can mitigate against being irrelevant to new research questions. While finger prick tests can be self-administered, a full venipuncture blood sample must be taken by medically trained personnel. Due to the need for medically trained personnel and the equipment required for refrigeration, transportation, storage, separation, processing, and analysis of samples, and potential long-term freezing for future testing, blood samples are more expensive than other biomarkers. Some blood biomarkers—for example, glucose, cholesterol, and cortisol levels—vary over the course of the day (Davis et al., 2023; Meier-Ewert et al., 2001). Therefore, the timing of when a blood sample is taken is important.

Blood is a key source of genetic and epigenetic biomarkers. These biomarkers are discussed in greater detail below in Box 7.2.

Box 7.2 Genetic and Epigenetic Biomarkers

DNA can be used to identify particular genes through genome-wide association studies (GWAS). These involve scanning markers across the genomes of many people to find genetic variations associated with a particular disease or condition. This may not be relevant to GUIDE now but could have potential for future research. More information may be found on the National Human Genome Research Institute.

Telomeres are nucleoprotein complexes of DNA sequences found at the end of chromosomes which protect against DNA damage during replication (McEachern et al., 2000; Verhoeven et al., 2024). While telomeres do shorten during replication as part of chronological aging, exposure to chronic stressors may accelerate telomere shortening due to oxidative stress and subsequent cellular damage (von Zglinicki, 2002). Recent research suggests that telomere length in adolescents is associated with environmental stress (Kertes et al., 2024).

Telomere length is a measure of cellular aging and declines with age. Due to this dynamism, studies have found that telomere length (TL) varies across different biospecimens. There is limited variation in TL across blood samples whose TL was significantly longer than buccal cells and saliva (Geronimus et al., 2021; Wolf et al., 2024). Therefore, care needs to be taken in selecting the best biospecimen.

The epigenome is made up of chemical compounds and proteins that can attach to DNA and direct such actions as turning genes on or off, controlling the production of proteins in particular cells (The National Human Genome Research Institute, 2020).

Environmental exposures, psychosocial stressors, and nutrition are all potentially important influences that may impact health outcomes directly or via interactions with the genome or epigenome over generations. Mounting evidence, primarily in animals, suggests that environmental exposures may generate or perpetuate altered health outcomes across one or more generations. One mechanism for these environmental health effects is via altered epigenetic regulation (Breton et al., 2021).

DNA methylation: physical and/or psychological stressors elicit a stress response which results in a cascade of downstream biological processes that can have implications on health. One commonly studied biological response to stress at the level of DNA is DNA methylation—a type of epigenetic process that influences gene expression by activating or inhibiting transcription. DNA methylation in children is investigated as an epigenetic measure of pace of biological aging and along with inflammation has been found to be associated with social inequalities and mental health in a recent twin study (Raffington et al., 2024; Salcedo-Bellido et al., 2021).

The sampling of dried blood spots (DBS) is routinely done for newborn babies. From DBS it is possible to examine hormone levels, exposure to tobacco, pesticides and some heavy metals, inflammatory cytokines, and DNA for genomic and epigenetic purposes (McClendon-Weary et al., 2020). If a biomarker exhibits diurnal variation (e.g., cortisol), repeated DBS would be more cost effective and less invasive than full blood sampling (McClendon-Weary et al., 2020).

Buccal Swabs

Buccal swabs gather epithelial cells from the lining of the mouth; they can be self-administered among older respondents and for infants and children collected via trained interviewers. DNA can be collected from buccal swabs, and these samples do not require refrigeration. Buccal swabs are a more cost-effective source of DNA/RNA than blood (Juárez-Cedillo et al., 2010).

Urine

Urine is produced by the kidneys filtering waste products from the blood; this waste is called urea. Urine, especially the first urine of the day, provides a range of biomarkers including hormones such as cortisol, metals from environmental exposure, and inflammatory markers, resulting for example from stress or infection. As Davis et al. (2023) discuss, urine can be collected in a range of ways: over 24 h, first morning samples, and spot collections. It degrades at room temperature; therefore, it is necessary to refrigerate or freeze samples. While possible in community settings, this does make urine difficult to collect, store, and transport and thus may not be the most feasible option to measure biomarkers in children.

Fecal Biome/Stools

At the time of writing it is understood that greater diversity and volume of fecal biome is associated with better health and therefore physical development. There is currently research into the relationship between fecal composition and the biome it contains (Vandeputte et al., 2016), which could eliminate the need for fecal samples and use photographs instead. It is plausible that in time data on fecal biome via photographs could replace a number of diet questions in surveys, thereby reducing participant burden. Collecting fecal material can be straightforward for babies but becomes more problematic for older children and adolescents in a community setting. National bowel cancer screening programs are testament to the viability of home collection and postal return methods for testing.

Other Health Data

Objective and Wider Health Data

At the most basic level, pedometers provide objective data on physical activity that could be included in GUIDE. They are relatively cheap devices and, if distributed to respondents in advance of a data collection wave, could measure the step counts of respondents and their main carer on defined days (e.g., Wednesday and Saturday), which could be entered via the online survey. The UK biobank uses cloud-enabled devices to collect this data. Many mobile phones and/or smart watches collect a range of data, including data on heart rate, sleep, social media usage, and physical activity. In terms of sleep and physical activity, mobile technology collects information on both quantity and quality of the activity. Data from mobile devices will be a valuable source of data when respondents reach the age of owning a phone. However, access to mobile phone data is subject to legislation of the country, and this applies to access to the data as first or third party, and review of data ownership, including with consumer-grade devices.

Linked Data

Linked data is routinely collected government data that can be "linked" to research data collected on individuals. Nordic countries provide excellent examples of using this opportunity; everyone has an individual identifier that enables researchers to link to data collected across government, health, education, and disease registries. Appendix C lists the linked data that has been included in the Growing up in Wales Study (Jones et al., 2024). Linked data collection costs are covered by other agencies, though matching linked data into GUIDE data will have a cost.

Environmental Indicators

A number of the cohorts surveyed collected air and dust samples at the household level.

Linked Environmental Data

Another way that linked data can be included is linking it geographically. National governments and the World Health Organization collect pollution data that is available to researchers. The UK Department for Environment, Farming, and Rural Affairs (DEFRA) has data available at the square kilometer level on ambient air quality, including anthropogenic particulate air pollution, available at local government area level. This data is available over time and could be incorporated into national GUIDE databases. Data on climactic pollution events could also be included, such as forest fires (e.g., in Greece) and flooding (e.g., in Valencia). With climate change being a key issue for young people, including these events and the proximity of individual homes to them will be key to assessing their impact on health and development, especially mental health.

In conclusion, selecting the appropriate biological indicators for a longitudinal cohort requires balancing scientific utility with logistical feasibility. While biological measures (such as anthropometry and lung function) provide essential baseline health data with relatively low burden, biospecimens offer deeper physiological insights into genetics, stress, and exposure—though they vary significantly in invasiveness and cost (e.g., the high yield but high resource requirement of blood versus the convenience of saliva or hair). Finally, other health data (including wearables and linked administrative records) presents a growing opportunity to capture objective environmental and lifestyle factors cost-effectively. Table 7.2 summarizes the pros and cons of different biological indicators in the context of a nationally representative population. Nationally representative samples by definition are not geographically focused and therefore clinic-based data collection would have to be set up by the research team, as happened for KiGGS (Mauz et al., 2020) and LSAC (Clifford et al., 2019).

Selection of Biological Indicators

The selection of biological indicators is influenced by four considerations: research themes to be examined, participant burden, ethical considerations, and costs.

Research Themes

Table 7.3 shows the research themes that can be examined via different biospecimens. In most cases the research theme dictates the timing of biological indicator collection. In a study examining healthy development up to age 25, physical development and activity levels would ideally be collected at each wave of data collection. Other measures are more complex: dental health could be measured at each wave, but it would be more cost effective to measure at the time of first primary tooth loss and last primary tooth loss, a difference of approximately 6 years. Environmental exposure should be measured for different periods of the life course—for example, preschool when exposure would predominantly be home or community based, compared to school age. Stress, as assessed by HPA axis activity, could be measured at key stages—for example pre-puberty, puberty, at the end of first year of high school, or at age 14 following 1 year of (legal) social media access.

Participant Burden

Participant burden is a key consideration in any research, but this is further amplified in the cumulative burden across successive waves within cohort studies and in studies that collect biological indicators. Studies with high participant burden suffer greater non-response and in the case of cohort studies are less likely to maintain high levels of respondent participation. Dietary data is a useful example to illustrate participant burden. Traditionally, dietary data is collected via survey questions. The complexity is evident when considering a simple consumption model: if five food groups are typically consumed over three daily meals, factoring in portion size, cooking method, snacks, and drinks, the required questions quickly exceed 30 per day. In one expert interview, Sean Cummings suggested that submitting photographs of food would reduce both participant burden and respondent recall errors. In another expert interview, Emmanuel Osimo stated that it will not be long before the fecal biome is a more reliable indicator of diet for some research questions.

Ulrich et al. (2018) list five levels of participant burden in clinical trials: physical, psychological, economic, familial, and societal. Data collection at the respondent's home or school places less burden on respondents and their caregivers. If data collection is in school, the burden is shifted. In the expert interview, Katy Shire from the Born in Bradford (BiB) cohort outlined the extensive staffing resources required to successfully initiate and maintain the engagement of schools. Recognizing that schools have little spare capacity, school participation in research needs to be at no cost (BiB paid £1000 to each school for administrative costs), be advantageous to the schools in terms of education opportunities and careers advice from the research team, and involve sharing results where practicable. BiB undertook class-based cognitive assessments, which were aggregated and shared with teachers and the results for study children were used in the research.

Table 7.3 Biological indicators by research themes

	Environmental exposure	Stress	Inflammation	Alcohol and drugs	Dental health	Physical development including puberty	Physical health
Biological measures							
Anthropometrics							
BP and pulse							
Physical activity							
Biospecimens							
Saliva							
Hair							
Nails							
Primary (baby) teeth							
Venous blood							
Dried blood spots							
Buccal swab							
Urine							
Fecal biome							
Other biological sampling							
Mite allergen/endotoxin in house dust							
Indoor gaseous atmospheric contaminants							
Linked data							
Health							
Environmental data							
Pollution							
Extreme weather events							

Biological indicators can be divided into 4 categories: excreta (feces and urine), bodily fluids and tissue (saliva, blood, and buccal swab), dead cells (hair, nails, and primary teeth) and measurements (height, weight, and activity level). The physical burden of collecting these samples is closely linked to which category it belongs to. Excreta need to be collected as they exit the body. Dead cells are routinely handled by respondents or their caregivers and often discarded (e.g., hair and primary teeth). Excreta and dead cells have limited physical burden. Bodily fluids or tissue are the most invasive group to be collected and therefore carry the greatest physical burden.

The measurement of height, weight, and activity level may not be physically invasive but can cause psychological distress: the fear of someone observing one's activity level or weight. Another psychological aspect is the disgust factor of saliva, excreta, or nail clippings. In MCS, it was found that this was overcome if children were allowed to go into another room to collect their saliva sample (Fitzsimons et al., 2022).

Ethical Considerations

While participant burden explicitly explores the impact of research design on participants, the ethical protocol protects an individual via voluntary participation, informed consent, the right to withdraw at any time, data processing that ensures confidentiality, and assessment that the benefits of the research outweigh the risks to participants (see Chap. 2 in this book).

Genetic data is considered "sensitive" under General Data Protection Regulation (GDPR), requiring greater protection than other measures mentioned in this chapter. This means that the consent procedure, collection, storage, and analysis of genetic data necessitate processes and procedures not required by other measures. One key aspect of genomic data is that it is time invariant, meaning it remains pertinent throughout an individual's lifetime. This raises several issues, including assent/consent, storage of samples, and access of the data. The age range of GUIDE is 0–25; if biological samples with time invariant indicators were taken with parental/carer consent, it would be advisable to attain respondent consent later. If biological samples are to be stored, it is extremely likely that theoretical and/or technological advances will result in this data being used for research questions unimagined at the time of data collection. Ethical procedures must accommodate these future developments and age-specific, religious, and cultural sensitivities.

The ethics of using data from mobile devices is complex. Use of this data is dependent on the legislation of the country where the data is generated, and participants can be unwilling to allow their data to be accessed due to concerns about geolocation.

Biospecimen Collection and Processing Costs

It is not straight forward to get publishable quotes for biospecimen processing; therefore, the following costs use the National Health Service (NHS) costs, online data on equipment and postage costs, estimates received for buccal swab collection, saliva and hair testing, and a dental research assistant for processing primary teeth for caries assessment. The cost for all biomarkers is beyond the scope of this chapter; for example, there are a total of 54 different inflammatory biomarkers (Dongiovanni et al., 2023). Where possible, the cost of single specific biomarkers is included. In Appendix D, where a web address is listed in the equipment, transport, and processing columns, this is a complete testing service either calculated by NICE or charged by a commercial company. Web addresses in a specific column indicate costs for that component of collection, for example collecting buccal cells.

Long-term biospecimen storage, the cost of incorporating results into the GUIDE database via bar codes, and researcher time are not included. A rough estimate of the cost of storing 40,000 EDTA (whole blood) samples would be £25,000 per annum. This is a clear example of where some biomarkers represent significant upfront investment for sampling and storage but can be justified by the future opportunity that it represents.

The variety of commercial sources included in Appendix D is noteworthy. These commercial sectors include private medical services, forensic science, and aesthetics, indicating the growing use of biological indicators by the UK population outside of the NHS.

Future Directions: Suggested GUIDE Biological Indicators

Table 7.4 shows the biological indicators suggested for the first 5 years of the GUIDE study to provide insight with children aged 8–12 and bearing in mind the aims and objectives, the research questions, participant burden, and cost. As biospecimens can provide multiple indicators, the figures indicate which biospecimen provides the measure. For example, primary teeth can provide measures of environmental exposure, but it is more cost effective and exposure appropriate to use hair for this measure. The indicators suggested are all self or carer reports, due to these being less burden for respondents/carers. Moreover, since the COVID 19 pandemic, self-sampling is more accepted. Consideration here of going beyond the first 5 years does not make sense because of academic and technical advances that will happen in the near future.

Table 7.4 Suggested biological indicators by research theme: cost per sample in GBP £

	Environmental exposure	Stress	Alcohol and drugs	Dental health	Physical development	Physical health	Unit costs
Height and Weight					25.95		25.95
Activity						6.79	6.79
Saliva							
Hair	88	45.89					133.89
Primary (baby) teeth				9.54			9.54
Total							176.05
Linked data							
Health							
Pollution							
Extreme weather events							

Hair

It is suggested that hair is collected to get a measure of HPA activity in the previous month. The cutting of hair is a relatively intrusive event for young people and therefore should be limited to pre-puberty (age 9) and puberty (age 12). Finally, collecting hair samples at the end of the summer term would allow hair to grow back during the holiday, reducing participant burden for some respondents.

Teeth

It is recommended that the first and last primary teeth are collected and classified for dental health. The collection of teeth is also a valuable opportunity for participant engagement opportunities to enhance cohort participation.

Height and Weight

By providing scales to each household, as in the Gemini study, the need for researchers to collect data is removed. It would be necessary to send batteries in advance of each data collection wave while also reminding respondents/carers to collect this data. Height data could be measured using a mobile phone, and both could then be inputted into the CAPI questionnaire. However, accuracy of the height measurements might be a problem.

Wearables

Similar to height and weight data, activity levels for the week or specific days preceding completion of the online survey should be requested, and this data should be entered into the online survey.

Environmental Linked Data

It is recommended that time series data on pollution and extreme weather events is incorporated into the GUIDE dataset.

Summary

The biological indicators recommended above are based on the framework for the selection of biological indicators proposed in this chapter. Data for five of the eight research themes is possible via the collection of only four samples: digital activity data, hair, primary teeth, and height/weight. These four samples are relatively non-invasive to collect, do not require participants to attend a clinic, and would cost a total of GBP £176.05 per participant to collect. The acceptability of collecting these and any future samples will have to be piloted. The most pertinent biological indicators will change over time and according to the age of GUIDE participants.

Future

Academic breakthroughs and technological developments in measuring biomarkers continue apace. As the GUIDE study develops, these breakthroughs and developments should be tracked so that GUIDE can take full advantage of biological indicators to increase our understanding of child and young person wellbeing and development.

Appendix A: Expert Consultation

We consulted with experts in the field of biological indicators of child and adolescent health to inform the content of this chapter. We include some specific reference to comments made but largely used the knowledge and expertise that they shared to direct our thinking. We would like to thank and acknowledge the time that the following experts afforded us:

Dr. Stephanie Cahill is currently a Quantitative Research Associate in the #BeeWell Program, Manchester Institute of Education. Dr. Cahill's PhD research aimed to investigate biosocial predictors of resilience to adverse childhood experiences, involving developing a quantitative methodology of measuring resilience across the life course using longitudinal birth cohort data. Delineating distinct trajectories of resilience using latent growth mixture modeling then using trajectory membership as phenotype in further genetic and epigenetic studies.

Dr. Andres Cardenas is Assistant Professor of Epidemiology at Stanford University (https://profiles.stanford.edu/Andres-Cardenas). Dr. Cardenas's research focuses on characterizing molecular and epigenetic biomarkers and the extent to which these alterations contribute to disease risk throughout the life course. His group utilizes computational approaches to investigate environmental chemical mixtures, biological aging markers, and fetal epigenetic programming.

Professor Sean Cumming at the University of Bath (https://researchportal.bath.ac.uk/en/persons/sean-cumming) is internationally recognized as a leading expert on the subject of growth and maturation in sport and exercise. Adopting a biocultural perspective, his research seeks to understand how biological and psychosocial factors impact athletic development and the maintenance of health behaviors during adolescence. He is highly experienced in the use of invasive and non-invasive methods for the assessment of growth and maturation in youth.

Professor Samantha Dockray, University College Cork (https://research.ucc.ie/profiles/s.dockray), has extensive experience in collecting biological samples for research on child and adolescent development, puberty, and allostatic load in studies conducted in five countries. She has led studies that collect blood, stool, urine, and saliva from adolescents, as well as studies that use wearable technologies to collect data on health-related behaviors, and health indicators such as heart rate variability. She incorporates patient-public involvement principles and activities to develop the design of studies that ask children and adolescents to provide biomarkers.

Meena Kumari is a professor at the University of Essex (https://www.iser.essex.ac.uk/people/mkumari). Kumari is a leading expert in biomarkers and genetics, and has worked to apply insights from these areas to better understand aging, cardiovascular disease, and health inequalities using the Whitehall II cohort study of British civil servants and the English Longitudinal Study of Ageing. Professor Kumari is the topic champion for health and biomarker content and research in Understanding Society and continues to lead research on the social-biological interface and genetic epidemiology as an investigator for the study.

Valeria Mondelli (https://kclpure.kcl.ac.uk/portal/en/persons/valeria.mondelli) is a Professor of Psychoneuroimmunology at the Institute of Psychiatry, Psychology, and Neuroscience at King's College London. She is an international expert in the study of blood- and saliva-based biomarkers in psychiatry. Her research focuses on the role of the biological stress response in the onset of mental health disorders and in the development of personalized interventions by using biomarker strategies. Prof Mondelli has co-led the international global mental health project Identifying Depression Early in Adolescence (IDEA project) which contributed to developing a risk score to identify adolescents at high risk of developing depression. She is Head of the PIXIE Lab (psychoneuroimmunometabolix and interaction with environment lab) and co-lead of the NIHR SLaM BRC Research Theme on Psychosis and Mood Disorders.

Dr. Emanuele Osimo (https://www.psychiatry.cam.ac.uk/staff/dr-emanuele-f-osimo) uses biomarkers and biological measures to inform research into developing clinically useful risk prediction models for psychiatric and physical health outcomes for the benefit of those with mental ill health.

Dr. Katy Shire (https://borninbradford.nhs.uk/about/our-team/dr-katy-shire/) is Program Manager for the BiB Age of Wonder program, which follows the BiB cohort through adolescence and into adulthood. This study involves biological samples including bloods at age 13–14 and age 18.

Appendix B

See Table 7.B1.

Appendix C

See Table 7.C1.

Appendix D

See Table 7.D1.

Table 7.B1 Cohort studies examined

	Geographical focus	n of bio sample types collected	Country	Date started	Survey sample size	Sampling for biological data	Location of biological data collection
ABCD (The Adolescent Brain Cognitive Development)	National	11	USA	2015	11,100	All	Clinic
Child cohort	National	10	Canada	‘08-’12	3297	All	Home/clinic
Etude Longitudinal Francaise depuis l’Enfance (ELFE)	National	5	France	2011	18,329	44% of maternity units	Home/clinic
Gemini: Health and development in twins	National	2	UK	2007	2402	All	Home
INMA	National	9	Spain	‘97-’08	3944	All	Clinic
Japan Environmental and children’s study	National	6	Japan	2011	100,148	Power calc	Clinic/ home
KIGGS[a]	National	10	Germany	2003	17,641	All in single wave	Clinic
Longitudinal study of Australian children (LSAC-CS)	National	15	Australia	2004	100,148	All in single wave	Clinic
Millenium birth cohort[b]	National	3	UK	2000	18,552	All in single wave	Home
MoBa	National	2	Norway	‘98-’06	114,000	All	Home
Born in Guangzhou Cohort Study (BIGCS)	Region	3	China	2012	17,214	All	Clinic
Baseline	Region	7	Ireland	2008	2137	All	Home/clinic
c-ABC	Region	5	China	2013	11,421	All, one city to adolescence	
GENV	Region	3	Australia	2021	120,000	All	Home
Odense child cohort	Region	3	Denmark	2010	2874	All	Home
Prospective Epidemiological Research studies in Iran Birth Cohort (PERSIAN)	Region	9	Iran	‘16-’17	Aim 15,000	All	Clinic
RHEA	Region	3	Greece	2007	1363	All	Home/clinic

(continued)

Table 7.B1 (continued)

	Geographical focus	n of bio sample types collected	Country	Date started	Survey sample size	Sampling for biological data	Location of biological data collection
Trials adolescent study	Region	4	Netherlands	2001	2230	All and clinical cohort	Clinic
Amsterdam Born Children and their Development (ABCD)	City	3	Netherlands	2003	8266 (bio 4389)	All	Home/school
Barcelona Life Study Cohort (BiSC)	City	7	Spain	2018	1032	All	Home/clinic
Born in Bradford	City	7	UK	2007	13,740		Home/school
The Copenhagen child cohort CCC2000	City	4	Denmark	2000	6090	All	Home
Determinants of Adolescent Social Wellbeing and Health (DASH)	City	5	UK	2003	6643	All	School
Eden	City	7	France	2003	1899	All	Clinic
Gateshead GMBS	City	5	UK	'99-'00	1029	All	Home/school
Generation R	City	10	Netherlands	2002	8305	<6YO sub sample. 6+ all	Clinic
Geracao XXI	City	9	Portugal	2005	8647	All	Home/clinic
REACH: resilience, ethnicity and adolescent mental health	City	1	UK	2016	4353	All	School
Southampton women's study	City	6	UK	'98-'02	2567	All and DXA subsample	Home
CHAMACOS	Community	6	USA	'99-'00	536	All	Home/community

[a] KIGGS undertook biological sampling in the original primary sampling unit (PSU) areas at wave 2 (age 10–29) in spite of awareness that a large number of respondents had by then moved to other areas. The KIGGS study made this decision based on the fact that it would be more cost effective to set up temporary clinics in 162 rather than all primary sampling units (PSU) in Germany

[b] The MCS was also advantaged, in the collection of biospecimens, by its original sampling frame in that it only had to send trained interviewers to specific local council wards

Table 7.C1 Linked electronic data available in Born in Wales

Sector	Dataset	Example variables
Demographics	Annual District Birth Extract (ADBE)	Place of birth
	ONS census Wales (CENW)	Ethnicity & household composition
	Welsh Demographic Service Dataset (WDSD)	Area deprivation score
Education	Education Wales (EDUW)	Attainment & free school meals
Health	Congenital Anomaly Register and Information Service (CARS)	ICD10 code
	COVID-19 vaccination and testing	Vaccination uptake
	Maternal Indicators Dataset (MIDS)	Apgar score
	Substance Misuse Dataset (SMDS)	Substance abuse problem
	National Community Child Health Database (NCCHD)	Birth weight
	Outpatient dataset for Wales (OPDW)	NHS hospital outpatient appointments
	Patient Episode Dataset for Wales (PEDW)	Hospital diagnoses & operations codes
	Welsh Longitudinal General Practice Dataset (WLGP)	Diagnoses & medications
	Welsh Study of Mothers and Babies (WOMBS)	Ultrasound scan for cognitive development
Welfare	Child Receiving Care and Support Census (CRCS)	On child protection register
	Child and Family Court Advisory and Support Service (CAFCASS)	Involved in family legal proceedings, divorces, family violence, etc.

Note Adapted from (Jones et al., 2024)

Table 7.D1 Collection and processing costs per sample

Biospecimen	Collection			Processing[1]	Biomarkers	Total
	Staff	Equipment	Transport			
Blood	NHS	NICE 2015			Full blood count	6.00
	Self/Parent	healthy.co			CRP	£39–£50
	At clinic	medichecks.com — Phoenix			CRP	£74–£80
	Nurse in home	medichecks.com — Phoenix			CRP	£98
Urine	NHS	NICE 2015			Urinalysis	£4.08
		NICE 2015			Dipstick	£3.85
Saliva			Refrigerated Post	£24.16 ARE	CRP	£25.81
	Self/parent	£1.65 ($2.08)		£28.71 ARE	IL-1β	£30.36
	Self/parent	£1.65 ($2.08)		£35.21 ARE	Cortisol	£36.86
		salimetrics.com				
					Methylation	
	Self/parent	the health society			Oral microbiome	£350

(continued)

[1] In this table processing is the cost of extracting the biomarker from biospecimen, e.g., cortisol from saliva or hair.

Table 7.D1 (continued)

Biospecimen	Collection			Processing	Biomarkers	Total
	Staff	Equipment	Transport			
Feces		Randox health			Microbiome	£190
	NHS bowel cancer screening unit cost	£5			Blood	£5
Dried blood spot		£3.30	£4.24		Cortisol RNA	
					Cholesterol	
Buccal swab	Self/parent	£1.88 Iso helix			RNA	
	Self/parent	dnatestingclinics.co.uk/			DNA for paternity testing	£99.00
		vie-aesthetics			Telomer	£455
		healthy.co			Methylation	£220
Hair	Interviewer, self or parent	£9.98		£35.90 ARE	Cortisol	45.89
	Self	mineral state			Single drug	£266

(continued)

Table 7.D1 (continued)

Biospecimen	Collection			Processing	Biomarkers	Total
	Staff	Equipment	Transport			
	At clinic	mineral state				£296
	Self	mineral state			9 drug panel	£511
	At clinic	mineral state				£541
	Self/parent	mineral state			7 heavy metals, 29 minerals	£88
Nails	Sent by parent	£3.69			DNA	
		AlphaBiolabs			DNA for relationship testing	£49
					Pollutants	
Teeth	Sent by parent	£4.54	3/hour research assistant	5.005	Caries	£9.54
					Heavy metals	
					Psychological distress	
Pedometer	Parent	£1.52	£5.27	n/a		£6.79
Axivity accelerometer	Parent	£129–139		n/a		£129–139
Scales	Parent	£22.00	£3.95	n/a	BMI	£25.95
Fingerprint	At pharmacy	dears pharmacy			Testing for 4 drug types	£49

Note ARE = Anglia Ruskin Enterprise

The NHS costs are lowest as they reflect the existing infrastructure, economies of scale, are pre- operative tests—in hospital not requiring transport and storage and date from 2015. The commercial costs are the highest estimates. Blood testing costs indicate the range within which research costs would lie £6–£98. The NHS unit cost for feces is from the bowel screening program. This is included to show that this is routinely collected in the UK and sent by post

The commercial buccal swab quotes show the expensive nature of epigenetic testing. The cost of hair tests indicates the viability of this biospecimen for cortisol and heavy metal mineral testing but not drug testing. The fingerprint testing for drugs would be a more cost-effective option. The variety of commercial sources included in Appendix 3 is noteworthy private medical providers. These commercial sectors include private medical services, forensic science, and aesthetics. Indicating the growing use of biological indicators by the UK population with the NHS

References

Benzeval, M. (2017, November). *Integrating biological and social science data: The experience of Understanding Society—The UK Household Longitudinal Survey* [Conference presentation]. *NCRM Autumn School 2017*, Southampton, United Kingdom. https://www.youtube.com/watch?v=SOY0G_1qu7I

Breton, C. V., Landon, R., Kahn, L. G., Enlow, M. B., Peterson, A. K., Bastain, T., ... & Fry, R. (2021). Exploring the evidence for epigenetic regulation of environmental influences on child health across generations. *Communications Biology, 4*(1), 769.

Bronfenbrenner, U., & Ceci, S. J. (1994). Nature-nurture reconceptualized in developmental perspective: A bioecological model. *Psychological Review, 101*(4), 568–586. https://doi.org/10.1037/0033-295X.101.4.568

Charles, M.-A., Thierry, X., Lanoe, J.-L., Bois, C., Dufourg, M.-N., Popa, R., Cheminat, M., Zaros, C., & Geay, B. (2020). Cohort profile: The French national cohort of children (ELFE): Birth to 5 years. *International Journal of Epidemiology, 49*(2), 368–369j. https://doi.org/10.1093/ije/dyz227

Clifford, S. A., Davies, S., Wake, M., & Child Health CheckPoint Team. (2019). Child Health CheckPoint: Cohort summary and methodology of a physical health and biospecimen module for the Longitudinal Study of Australian Children. *BMJ Open, 9*(Suppl 3), 3–22. https://doi.org/10.1136/bmjopen-2017-020261

Cole, T. J. (2018). Optimal design for longitudinal studies to estimate pubertal height growth in individuals. *Annals of Human Biology, 45*(4), 314–320.

Currie, C., & Morgan, A. (2020). A bio-ecological framing of evidence on the determinants of adolescent mental health: A scoping review of the international Health Behaviour in School-Aged Children (HBSC) study 1983–2020. *SSM—Population Health, 12*, Article 100697. https://doi.org/10.1016/j.ssmph.2020.100697

Currie, C., & Morgan, A. (2024). *Conceptualising sustainable child and adolescent health: A bio-ecological framework*. OSF Preprints. https://doi.org/10.31219/osf.io/eyk52

Davis, S. L., Latimer, M., & Rice, M. (2023). Biomarkers of stress and inflammation in children. *Biological Research for Nursing, 25*(4), 559–570. https://doi.org/10.1177/10998004231168805

Dongiovanni, P., Meroni, M., Casati, S., Goldoni, R., Thomaz, D. V., Kehr, N. S., Galimberti, D., Del Fabbro, M., & Tartaglia, G. M. (2023). Salivary biomarkers: Novel noninvasive tools to diagnose chronic inflammation. *International Journal of Oral Science, 15*(1), Article 27. https://doi.org/10.1038/s41368-023-00231-6

Drosopoulou, G., Sergentanis, T. N., Mastorakos, G., Vlachopapadopoulou, E., Michalacos, S., Tzavara, C., Bacopoulou, F., Psaltopoulou, T., & Tsitsika, A. (2021). Psychosocial health of adolescents in relation to underweight, overweight/obese status: The EU NET ADB survey. *European Journal of Public Health, 31*(2), 379–384. https://doi.org/10.1093/eurpub/ckaa189

Eriksen, C., Boustedt, K., Sonne, S. B., Dahlgren, J., Kristiansen, K., Twetman, S., Brix, S., & Roswall, J. (2024). Early life factors and oral microbial signatures define the risk of caries in a Swedish cohort of preschool children. *Scientific Reports, 14*(1), Article 8463. https://doi.org/10.1038/s41598-024-59126-z

Fitzsimons, E., Moulton, V., Hughes, D. A., Neaves, S., Ho, K., Hemani, G., Timpson, N., Calderwood, L., Gilbert, E., & Ring, S. (2022). Collection of genetic data at scale for a nationally representative population: The UK Millennium Cohort Study. *Longitudinal and Life Course Studies, 13*(1), 169–187. https://doi.org/10.1332/175795921X16223668101602

Fraser, A., Macdonald-Wallis, C., Tilling, K., Boyd, A., Golding, J., Davey Smith, G., Henderson, J., Macleod, J., Molloy, L., Ness, A., Ring, S., Nelson, S. M., & Lawlor, D. A. (2013). Cohort profile: The Avon Longitudinal Study of Parents and Children: ALSPAC mothers cohort. *International Journal of Epidemiology, 42*(1), 97–110. https://doi.org/10.1093/ije/dys066

Garrido-Miguel, M., Martínez-Vizcaíno, V., Oliveira, A., Martínez-Andrés, M., Sequí-Domínguez, I., Hernández-Castillejo, L. E., & Cavero-Redondo, I. (2021). Prevalence and trends of underweight in European children and adolescents: A systematic review and meta-analysis. *European Journal of Nutrition, 60*(7), 3611–3624. https://doi.org/10.1007/s00394-021-02540-0

Geronimus, A. T., Bound, J., Mitchell, C., Martinez-Cardoso, A., Evans, L., Hughes, L., Schneper, L., & Notterman, D. A. (2021). Coming up short: Comparing venous blood, dried blood spots & saliva samples for measuring telomere length in health equity research. *PLOS ONE, 16*(8), Article e0255237. https://doi.org/10.1371/journal.pone.0255237

Gomez, A., & Nelson, K. E. (2017). The oral microbiome of children: Development, disease, and implications beyond oral health. *Microbial Ecology, 73*(2), 492–503. https://doi.org/10.1007/s00248-016-0854-1

Huang, T., Howse, F. M., Stachenfeld, N. S., & Usselman, C. W. (2023). Correlations between salivary- and blood-derived gonadal hormone assessments and implications for inclusion of female participants in research studies. *American Journal of Physiology-Heart and Circulatory Physiology, 324*(1), H33–H46. https://doi.org/10.1152/ajpheart.00399.2022

Jaddoe, V. W. V., Mackenbach, J. P., Moll, H. A., Steegers, E. A. P., Tiemeier, H., Verhulst, F. C., Witteman, J. C. M., & Hofman, A. (2006). The Generation R Study: Design and cohort profile. *European Journal of Epidemiology, 21*(6), 475–484. https://doi.org/10.1007/s10654-006-9022-0

Jebeile, H., Kelly, A. S., O'Malley, G., & Baur, L. A. (2022). Obesity in children and adolescents: Epidemiology, causes, assessment, and management. *The Lancet Diabetes & Endocrinology, 10*(5), 351–365. https://doi.org/10.1016/S2213-8587(22)00047-X

Jones, H., Seaborne, M. J., Kennedy, N. L., James, M., Dredge, S., Bandyopadhyay, A., Battaglia, A., Davies, S., & Brophy, S. (2024). Cohort profile: Born in Wales—A birth cohort with maternity, parental and child data linkage for life course research in Wales, UK. *BMJ Open, 14*(1), Article e076711. https://doi.org/10.1136/bmjopen-2023-076711

Juárez-Cedillo, T., Sánchez-García, S., Mould-Quevedo, J. F., García-Peña, C., Gallo, J. J., Wagner, F. A., & Vargas-Alarcón, G. (2010). Cost-effective analysis of genotyping using oral cells in the geriatric population. *Genetics and Molecular Research, 9*(3), 1886–1895. https://doi.org/10.4238/vol9-3gmr939

Kertes, D. A., Clendinen, C., Duan, K., Rabinowitz, J. A., Browning, C., & Kvam, P. (2024). The social environment matters for telomere length and internalizing problems during adolescence. *Journal of Youth and Adolescence, 53*(1), 21–35. https://doi.org/10.1007/s10964-023-01848-w

Mauz, E., Lange, M., Houben, R., Hoffmann, R., Allen, J., Gößwald, A., Hölling, H., Lampert, T., Lange, C., Poethko-Müller, C., Richter, A., Schaffrath Rosario, A., von Schenck, U., Ziese, T., Kurth, B.-M., & KiGGS Cohort Research Team. (2020). Cohort profile: KiGGS cohort longitudinal study on the health of children, adolescents and young adults in Germany. *International Journal of Epidemiology, 49*(2), 375–375k. https://doi.org/10.1093/ije/dyz231

McClendon-Weary, B., Putnick, D. L., Robinson, S., & Yeung, E. (2020). Little to give, much to gain—what can you do with a dried blood spot? *Current Environmental Health Reports, 7*(3), 211–221.

McEachern, M. J., Krauskopf, A., & Blackburn, E. H. (2000). Telomeres and their control. *Annual Review of Genetics, 34*(1), 331–358. https://doi.org/10.1146/annurev.genet.34.1.331

Meier-Ewert, H. K., Ridker, P. M., Rifai, N., Price, N., Dinges, D. F., & Mullington, J. M. (2001). Absence of diurnal variation of C-reactive protein concentrations in healthy human subjects. *Clinical Chemistry, 47*(3), 426–430.

Michikawa, T., Nitta, H., Nakayama, S. F., Ono, M., Yonemoto, J., Tamura, K., Suda, E., Ito, H., Takeuchi, A., & Kawamoto, T. (2015). The Japan Environment and Children's Study (JECS): A preliminary report on selected characteristics of approximately 10,000 pregnant women recruited during the first year of the study. *Journal of Epidemiology, 25*(6), 452–458. https://doi.org/10.2188/jea.JE20140186

National Human Genome Research Institute. (2020, August 17). *Genome-wide association studies fact sheet*. https://www.genome.gov/about-genomics/fact-sheets/Genome-Wide-Association-Studies-Fact-Sheet

Omary, A., Curtis, M., Cheng, T. W., Mair, P., Shirtcliff, E. A., Barch, D. M., & Somerville, L. H. (2025). Multimodal measurement of pubertal development: stage, timing, tempo, and hormones. *Child Develop, 96*(3), 980–999.

Ortega, F. B., Leskošek, B., Blagus, R., Gil-Cosano, J. J., Mäestu, J., Tomkinson, G. R., Ruiz, J. R., Mäestu, E., Starc, G., Milanović, I., Tammelin, T. H., Sorić, M., Scheuer, C., Carraro, A., Kaj, M., Csányi, T., Sardinha, L. B., Lenoir, M., Emeljanovas, A., ... Jurak, G. (2023). European fitness landscape for children and adolescents: Updated reference values, fitness maps and country rankings based on nearly 8 million test results from 34 countries gathered by the FitBack network. *British Journal of Sports Medicine, 57*(5), 299–310. https://doi.org/10.1136/bjsports-2022-106176

Poulton, R., Moffitt, T. E., & Silva, P. A. (2015). The Dunedin Multidisciplinary Health and Development Study: Overview of the first 40 years, with an eye to the future. *Social Psychiatry and Psychiatric Epidemiology, 50*(5), 679–693. https://doi.org/10.1007/s00127-015-1048-8

Raffington, L., Tanksley, P. T., Vinnik, L., Sabhlok, A., Patterson, M. W., Mallard, T., Malanchini, M., Ayorech, Z., Tucker-Drob, E. M., & Paige Harden, K. (2024). Associations of DNA-methylation measures of biological aging with social disparities in child and adolescent mental health. *Clinical Psychological Science, 12*(4), 551–562. https://doi.org/10.1177/21677026231186802

Regulation (EU) 2016/679 of the European Parliament and of the Council of 27 April 2016 on the protection of natural persons with regard to the processing of personal data and on the free movement of such data, and repealing Directive 95/46/EC (General Data Protection Regulation). (2016). *Official Journal of the European Union, L 119*, 1–88. https://eur-lex.europa.eu/eli/reg/2016/679/oj

Salcedo-Bellido, I., Gutiérrez-González, E., García-Esquinas, E., Fernández de Larrea-Baz, N., Navas-Acien, A., Téllez-Plaza, M., Pastor-Barriuso, R., Lope, V., Gómez-Ariza, J. L., García-Barrera, T., Pollán, M., Jiménez Moleón, J. J., & Pérez-Gómez, B. (2021). Toxic metals in toenails as biomarkers of exposure: A review. *Environmental Research, 197*, Article 111028. https://doi.org/10.1016/j.envres.2021.111028

Ulrich, C. M., Zhou, Q., Ratcliffe, S. J., Knafl, K., Wallen, G. R., Richmond, T. S., & Grady, C. (2018). Development and preliminary testing of the perceived benefit and burden scales for cancer clinical trial participation. *Journal of Empirical Research on Human Research Ethics, 13*(3), 230–238.

Vandeputte, D., Falony, G., Vieira-Silva, S., Tito, R. Y., Joossens, M., & Raes, J. (2016). Stool consistency is strongly associated with gut microbiota richness and composition, enterotypes and bacterial growth rates. *Gut, 65*(1), 57–62. https://doi.org/10.1136/gutjnl-2015-309618

Verhoeven, J. E., Wolkowitz, O. M., Barr Satz, I., Conklin, Q., Lamers, F., Lavebratt, C., Lin, J., Lindqvist, D., Mayer, S. E., Melas, P. A., Milaneschi, Y., Picard, M., Rampersaud, R., Rasgon, N., Ridout, K., Söderberg Veibäck, G., Trumpff, C., Tyrka, A. R., Watson, K., ... Han, L. K. M. (2024). The researcher's guide to selecting biomarkers in mental health studies. *BioEssays, 46*(10), 2300246. https://doi.org/10.1002/bies.202300246

von Zglinicki, T. (2002). Oxidative stress shortens telomeres. *Trends in Biochemical Sciences, 27*(7), 339–344. https://doi.org/10.1016/S0968-0004(02)02110-2

Wolf, S. E., Hastings, W. J., Ye, Q., Etzel, L., Apsley, A. T., Chiaro, C., Heim, C. C., Heller, T., Noll, J. G., & Schreier, H. M. C. (2024). Cross-tissue comparison of telomere length and quality metrics of DNA among individuals aged 8 to 70 years. *PLoS ONE, 19*(2), e0290918. https://doi.org/10.1371/journal.pone.0290918

Wright, J., Small, N., Raynor, P., Tuffnell, D., Bhopal, R., Cameron, N., Fairley, L., Lawlor, D. A., Parslow, R., Petherick, E. S., Pickett, K. E., Waiblinger, D., West, J., & Born in Bradford Scientific Collaborators Group. (2013). Cohort profile: The Born in Bradford multi-ethnic family cohort study. *International Journal of Epidemiology, 42*(4), 978–991. https://doi.org/10.1093/ije/dys112

Cohort Study References

Amorim, M., Soares, S., Abrahamyan, A., Severo, M., & Fraga, S. (2023). Patterns of childhood adversity and health outcomes in early adolescence: Results from the Generation XXI cohort. *Preventive Medicine, 171*, Article 107500. https://doi.org/10.1016/j.ypmed.2023.107500

Bagot, K. S., Matthews, S. A., Mason, M., Squeglia, L. M., Fowler, J., Gray, K., Herting, M., May, A., Colrain, I., Godino, J., Tapert, S., Brown, S., & Patrick, K. (2018). Current, future and potential use of mobile and wearable technologies and social media data in the ABCD study to increase understanding of contributors to child health. *Developmental Cognitive Neuroscience, 32*, 121–129. https://doi.org/10.1016/j.dcn.2018.03.008

Chatzi, L., Leventakou, V., Vafeiadi, M., Koutra, K., Roumeliotaki, T., Chalkiadaki, G., Karachaliou, M., Daraki, V., Kyriklaki, A., Kampouri, M., Fthenou, E., Sarri, K., Vassilaki, M., Fasoulaki, M., Bitsios, P., Koutis, A., Stephanou, E. G., & Kogevinas, M. (2017). Cohort profile: The mother-child cohort in Crete, Greece (Rhea Study). *International Journal of Epidemiology, 46*(5), 1392–1393k. https://doi.org/10.1093/ije/dyx084

Connelly, R., & Platt, L. (2014). Cohort profile: UK Millennium Cohort Study (MCS). *International Journal of Epidemiology, 43*(6), 1719–1725. https://doi.org/10.1093/ije/dyu001

Dadvand, P., Gascon, M., Bustamante, M., Rivas, I., Foraster, M., Basagaña, X., Cosín, M., Eixarch, E., Ferrer, M., Gratacós, E., Gómez Herrera, L., Jimenez-Arenas, P., Júlvez, J., Morillas, À., Nieuwenhuijsen, M. J., Persavento, C., Pujol, J., Querol, X., Sánchez García, O., ... BiSC Group. (2024). Cohort profile: Barcelona life study cohort (BiSC). *International Journal of Epidemiology, 53*(3), Article dyae063. https://doi.org/10.1093/ije/dyae063

Dick, A. S., Lopez, D. A., Watts, A. L., Heeringa, S., Reuter, C., Bartsch, H., Fan, C. C., Kennedy, D. N., Palmer, C., Marshall, A., Haist, F., Hawes, S., Nichols, T. E., Barch, D. M., Jernigan, T. L., Garavan, H., Grant, S., Pariyadath, V., Hoffman, E., ... Thompson, W. K. (2021). Meaningful associations in the Adolescent Brain Cognitive Development study. *NeuroImage, 239*, Article 118262. https://doi.org/10.1016/j.neuroimage.2021.118262

Granados, A., Gebremariam, A., & Lee, J. M. (2015). Relationship between timing of peak height velocity and pubertal staging in boys and girls. *Journal of Clinical Research in Pediatric Endocrinology, 7*(3), 235.

Guxens, M., Ballester, F., Espada, M., Fernández, M. F., Grimalt, J. O., Ibarluzea, J., Olea, N., Rebagliato, M., Tardón, A., Torrent, M., Vioque, J., Vrijheid, M., Sunyer, J., & INMA Project. (2012). Cohort profile: The INMA—INfancia y Medio Ambiente—(Environment and Childhood) Project. *International Journal of Epidemiology, 41*(4), 930–940. https://doi.org/10.1093/ije/dyr054

Harding, S., Whitrow, M., Maynard, M. J., & Teyhan, A. (2007). Cohort profile: The DASH (determinants of adolescent social well-being and health) study, an ethnically diverse cohort. *International Journal of Epidemiology, 36*(3), 512–517. https://doi.org/10.1093/ije/dym094

Heude, B., Forhan, A., Slama, R., Douhaud, L., Bedel, S., Saurel-Cubizolles, M.-J., Hankard, R., Thiebaugeorges, O., de Agostini, M., Annesi-Maesano, I., Kaminski, M., & Charles, M.-A. (2016). Cohort profile: The EDEN mother-child cohort on the prenatal and early postnatal determinants of child health and development. *International Journal of Epidemiology, 45*(2), 353–363. https://doi.org/10.1093/ije/dyv151

Hoffmann, R., Lange, M., Butschalowsky, H., Houben, R., Schmich, P., Allen, J., Kuhnert, R., Rosario, A. S., & Gößwald, A. (2018). KiGGS Wave 2 cross-sectional study—Participant acquisition, response rates and representativeness. *Journal of Health Monitoring, 3*(1), 78–91. https://doi.org/10.17886/RKI-GBE-2018-032

Huisman, M., Oldehinkel, A. J., de Winter, A., Minderaa, R. B., de Bildt, A., Huizink, A. C., Verhulst, F. C., & Ormel, J. (2008). Cohort profile: The Dutch 'TRacking Adolescents' Individual Lives' Survey'; TRAILS. *International Journal of Epidemiology, 37*(6), 1227–1235. https://doi.org/10.1093/ije/dym273

Inskip, H. M., Godfrey, K. M., Robinson, S. M., Law, C. M., Barker, D. J. P., & Cooper, C. (2006). Cohort profile: The Southampton Women's Survey. *International Journal of Epidemiology, 35*(1), 42–48. https://doi.org/10.1093/ije/dyi202

Jaddoe, V. W. V., Bakker, R., van Duijn, C. M., van der Heijden, A. J., Lindemans, J., Mackenbach, J. P., Moll, H. A., Steegers, E. A. P., Tiemeier, H., Uitterlinden, A. G., Verhulst, F. C., & Hofman, A. (2007). The Generation R Study Biobank: A resource for epidemiological studies in children and their parents. *European Journal of Epidemiology, 22*(12), 917–923. https://doi.org/10.1007/s10654-007-9209-z

Knowles, G., Gayer-Anderson, C., Blakey, R., Davis, S., Lowis, K., Stanyon, D., Ofori, A., Turner, A., Dorn, L., Schools Working Group, Young Persons Advisory Group, Beards, S., Pinfold, V., Reininghaus, U., Harding, S., & Morgan, C. (2022). Cohort profile: Resilience, Ethnicity and AdolesCent mental Health (REACH). *International Journal of Epidemiology, 51*(5), e303–e313. https://doi.org/10.1093/ije/dyac051

Kyhl, H. B., Jensen, T. K., Barington, T., Buhl, S., Norberg, L. A., Jørgensen, J. S., Jensen, D. F. G., Christesen, H. T., Lamont, R. F., & Husby, S. (2015). The Odense Child Cohort: Aims, design, and cohort profile. *Paediatric and Perinatal Epidemiology, 29*(3), 250–258. https://doi.org/10.1111/ppe.12183

Magnus, P., Birke, C., Vejrup, K., Haugan, A., Alsaker, E., Daltveit, A. K., Handal, M., Haugen, M., Høiseth, G., Knudsen, G. P., Magnus, M. C., Stoltenberg, C., Surén, P., Vold, L., & Stoltenberg, C. (2016). Cohort profile update: The Norwegian Mother and Child Cohort Study (MoBa). *International Journal of Epidemiology, 45*(2), 382–388. https://doi.org/10.1093/ije/dyw029

Magnus, P., Irgens, L. M., Haug, K., Nystad, W., Skjærven, R., Stoltenberg, C., & The MoBa Study Group. (2006). Cohort profile: The Norwegian Mother and Child Cohort Study (MoBa). *International Journal of Epidemiology, 35*(5), 1146–1150. https://doi.org/10.1093/ije/dyl170

Mauz, E., Lange, M., Houben, R., Hoffmann, R., Allen, J., Gößwald, A., Hölling, H., Lampert, T., Lange, C., Poethko-Müller, C., Richter, A., Schaffrath Rosario, A., von Schenck, U., Ziese, T., Kurth, B.-M., & on behalf of the KiGGS Cohort Research Team. (2020). Cohort profile: KiGGS cohort longitudinal study on the health of children, adolescents and young adults in Germany. *International Journal of Epidemiology, 49*(2), 375–375k. https://doi.org/10.1093/ije/dyz231

McEachan, R. R. C., Santorelli, G., Watmuff, A., Mason, D., Barber, S. E., Bingham, D. D., Bird, P. K., Lennon, L., Lewer, D., Mon-Williams, M., Shire, K. A., Waiblinger, D., West, J., Yang, T. C., Lawlor, D. A., Pickett, K. E., & Wright, J. (2024). Cohort profile update: Born in Bradford. *International Journal of Epidemiology, 53*(2), Article dyae037. https://doi.org/10.1093/ije/dyae037

O'Donovan, S. M., Murray, D. M., Hourihane, J. O. B., Kenny, L. C., Irvine, A. D., & Kiely, M. (2015). Cohort profile: The Cork BASELINE Birth Cohort Study: Babies after SCOPE: Evaluating the longitudinal impact on neurological and nutritional endpoints. *International Journal of Epidemiology, 44*(3), 764–775. https://doi.org/10.1093/ije/dyu157

Oldehinkel, A. J., Rosmalen, J. G. M., Buitelaar, J. K., Hoek, H. W., Ormel, J., Raven, D., Reijneveld, S. A., Veenstra, R., Verhulst, F. C., Vollebergh, W. A. M., & Hartman, C. A. (2015). Cohort profile update: The Tracking Adolescents' Individual Lives Survey (TRAILS). *International Journal of Epidemiology, 44*(1), 76–76n. https://doi.org/10.1093/ije/dyu225

Olsen, E. M., Rask, C. U., Elberling, H., Jeppesen, P., Clemmensen, L., Munkholm, A., Li, X.-Q., Hansen, M. H., Rimvall, M. K., & Linneberg, A. (2020). Cohort profile: The Copenhagen Child Cohort Study (CCC2000). *International Journal of Epidemiology, 49*(2), 370–371l. https://doi.org/10.1093/ije/dyz256

Parkinson, K. N., Pearce, M. S., Dale, A., Reilly, J. J., Drewett, R. F., Wright, C. M., Relton, C. L., McArdle, P., Le Couteur, A. S., & Adamson, A. J. (2011). Cohort profile: The Gateshead Millennium Study. *International Journal of Epidemiology, 40*(2), 308–317. https://doi.org/10.1093/ije/dyq015

Qiu, X., Lu, J.-H., He, J.-R., Lam, K. H., Shen, S.-Y., Guo, Y., Kuang, Y.-S., Yuan, M.-Y., Qiu, L., Chen, N.-N., Lu, M.-S., Li, W.-D., Xing, Y.-F., Bartington, S., Zhou, F.-J., Cheng, K. K., &

Xia, H.-M. (2017). The Born in Guangzhou Cohort Study (BIGCS). *European Journal of Epidemiology, 32*(4), 337–346. https://doi.org/10.1007/s10654-017-0239-x

Sekiyama, M., Yamazaki, S., Michikawa, T., Nakayama, S. F., Nitta, H., Taniguchi, Y., Suda, E., Isobe, T., Kobayashi, Y., & Iwai-Shimada, M. (2022). Study design and participants' profile in the sub-cohort study in the Japan Environment and Children's Study (JECS). *Journal of Epidemiology, 32*(5), 228–236. https://doi.org/10.2188/jea.JE20200448

Takaro, T. K., Scott, J. A., Allen, R. W., Anand, S. S., Becker, A. B., Befus, A. D., Brauer, M., Duncan, J. M., Lefebvre, D. L., Lou, W. Y. W., Mandhane, P. J., McLean, K. E., Miller, G., Sbihi, H., Shu, H., Subbarao, P., Turvey, S. E., Wheeler, A. J., Zeng, L., ... The CHILD study investigators. (2015). The Canadian Healthy Infant Longitudinal Development (CHILD) birth cohort study: Assessment of environmental exposures. *Journal of Exposure Science & Environmental Epidemiology, 25*(6), 580–592. https://doi.org/10.1038/jes.2015.7

Tao, F.-B., Hao, J.-H., Huang, K., Su, P.-Y., Cheng, D.-J., Xing, X.-Y., Huang, Z.-H., Zhang, J.-L., & Tong, S.-L. (2013). Cohort profile: The China-Anhui birth cohort study. *International Journal of Epidemiology, 42*(3), 709–721. https://doi.org/10.1093/ije/dys085

Uban, K. A., Horton, M. K., Jacobus, J., Heyser, C., Thompson, W. K., Tapert, S. F., Madden, P. A. F., & Sowell, E. R. (2018). Biospecimens and the ABCD study: Rationale, methods of collection, measurement and early data. *Developmental Cognitive Neuroscience, 32*, 97–106. https://doi.org/10.1016/j.dcn.2018.03.005

van Eijsden, M., Vrijkotte, T. G. M., Gemke, R. J. B. J., & van der Wal, M. F. (2011). Cohort profile: The Amsterdam Born Children and their Development (ABCD) study. *International Journal of Epidemiology, 40*(5), 1176–1186. https://doi.org/10.1093/ije/dyq128

van Jaarsveld, C. H. M., Johnson, L., Llewellyn, C., & Wardle, J. (2010). Gemini: A UK twin birth cohort with a focus on early childhood weight trajectories, appetite and the family environment. *Twin Research and Human Genetics, 13*(1), 72–78. https://doi.org/10.1375/twin.13.1.72

Vernet, C., Johnson, M., Kogut, K., Hyland, C., Deardorff, J., Bradman, A., & Eskenazi, B. (2021). Organophosphate pesticide exposure during pregnancy and childhood and onset of juvenile delinquency by age 16 years: The CHAMACOS cohort. *Environmental Research, 197*, Article 111055. https://doi.org/10.1016/j.envres.2021.111055

Wake, M., Goldfeld, S., Mohal, J., Siero, W., Hughes, E., Clifford, S., Hall, S., Schwarz, N., Frugier, T., Wang, J., Mavoa, S., Zaritski, N., & Saffery, R. (2024). Generation Victoria (GenV): Creating a large consented longitudinal infrastructure for discovery and intervention research. *International Journal of Population Data Science, 9*(5), 329. https://doi.org/10.23889/ijpds.v9i5.2822

Wright, J., Small, N., Raynor, P., Tuffnell, D., Bhopal, R., Cameron, N., Fairley, L., Lawlor, D. A., Parslow, R., Petherick, E. S., Pickett, K. E., Waiblinger, D., West, J., & on behalf of the Born in Bradford Scientific Collaborators Group. (2013). Cohort profile: The Born in Bradford multi-ethnic family cohort study. *International Journal of Epidemiology, 42*(4), 978–991. https://doi.org/10.1093/ije/dys112

Zare Sakhvidi, M. J., Danaei, N., Dadvand, P., Mehrparvar, A. H., Heidari-Beni, M., Nouripour, S., Nikukar, H., Daniali, S. S., Saffarieh, E., Noorishadkam, M., Amin, M. M., Mirmohammadkhani, M., Lotfi, M. H., Vaez, A., Mirmohammadi, S. J., Zarean, E., Mojibian, M., Hashemipour, M., Yaghini, O., ... Kelishadi, R. (2021). The prospective epidemiological research studies in IrAN (PERSIAN) birth cohort protocol: Rationale, design and methodology. *Longitudinal and Life Course Studies, 12*(2), 241–262. https://doi.org/10.1332/175795920X16062247639874

Candace Currie (Ph.D.) is an honorary professor at University College London. She has previously held personal chairs in Child and Adolescent Health at the Universities of Edinburgh and St Andrews, where she established the Child and Adolescent Health Research Unit (CAHRU) in 2000. Her research focuses on socioeconomic and gender inequalities, as well as pubertal development and its impact on adolescent health and wellbeing.

Juliet McEachran (Ph.D.) is a social scientist holding a doctorate in Demography. She has worked in academia, the third sector, and for the World Health Organization. Her career focuses on utilizing evidence to leverage change.

Chapter 8
Open Science in Longitudinal, Cohort Designs with Children

Diana Zavala-Rojas and Hannah Schwarz

Introduction

In 2016, there were two paradigm shifts in the approach to data in Europe. On the one hand, the Findable-Accessible-Interoperable-Reusable (FAIR) data principles were published to provide a technical framework for data to comply with Open Science. On the other hand, the General Data Protection Regulation (GDPR) was adopted. With this, the terms data governance, data stewardship and data management became part of the day-to-day jargon across all scientific domains. As a consequence, survey projects, including those having children as their main participants, had to expand their practices in data protection, data archiving, and data access to comply with both FAIR and GDPR.

Open Science, FAIR, and GDPR are legally binding frameworks to EU publicly funded scientific projects using human data (European Commission, Directorate-General for Research and Innovation, 2021). These frameworks have become pillars of science policy. While Open Science has different definitions and interpretations (Vicente-Saez & Martínez-Fuentes, 2018), in this chapter we use the definition by the European Commission as "an approach to research based on open cooperative work that emphasizes the sharing of knowledge, results and tools as early and widely as possible" (European Commission, 2024). Open Science policy in Europe rests on eight principles: FAIR Data, Research Integrity, Next Generation Metrics, Future of Scholarly Communication, Citizen Science, Education and Skills, a system of Open Science Rewards and Incentives, and the European Open Science Cloud (European Commission, Directorate-General for Research and Innovation, 2019, 2021). In

D. Zavala-Rojas (✉) · H. Schwarz
Department of Political and Social Sciences, Universitat Pompeu Fabra, Barcelona, Spain
e-mail: diana.zavala@upf.edu

D. Zavala-Rojas
European Social Survey ERIC, City St George's, University of London, London, United Kingdom

L. K. Taylor et al. (eds.), *Growing Up in Digital Europe*, Springer Series on Child and Family Studies, https://doi.org/10.1007/978-3-032-30592-3_8

short, Open Science is mandatory under Horizon Europe, and it operates on the principle of being as open as possible and as closed as necessary (European Commission, 2024). In this chapter, we focus on the FAIR component of Open Science because it offers a starting point for the technical implementation of Open Science. FAIR is a component that should be endorsed by Research Infrastructures (data stewards) in order for researchers and data users to achieve Open Science; therefore, our aim in this chapter is to provide a set of recommendations for Growing Up in Digital Europe (GUIDE) to commit to the highest standards of FAIR but also data protection at the same time.

FAIR provides technical guidelines that contribute to the openness of data-driven science (Wilkinson et al., 2016) by allowing the Findability of data and metadata based on unique identifiers; supplying Accessibility by stipulating protocols in which metadata would continue in existence, even in cases when the data itself were no longer available; enhancing data Interoperability, in which data and metadata are compatible with a wide range of applications to facilitate the analysis, storage, and processing of data; and promoting the Reuse of digital assets, dependent on the accurate and clear description of the data and metadata licensing.

For some, FAIR and GDPR contradict each other: GDPR is seen as a barrier, restricting and counteracting open sharing of personal data (Ursin & Bentzen, 2021). For others, they complement each other: data protection sets the legal boundaries for unrestricted openness of human data collected for the purposes of research (Phillips & Knoppers, 2019). While this debate is ongoing, there is a necessity for emerging and consolidated projects collecting human data to find a practical way to comply with both FAIR and GDPR.

The next section outlines potential tensions between implementing the FAIR framework and advancing data protection in line with the GDPR. We then present four European longitudinal surveys with children, highlighting their practices, best approaches, and challenges, including age thresholds for informed consent. This is followed by an overview of good FAIR practices in the Survey of Health, Ageing and Retirement in Europe (SHARE), a longitudinal study of people aged 50 and above. Finally, rooted in this literature review, we offer recommendations for GUIDE to consider that could potentially strengthen Open Science and data protection.[1]

Potential Tensions and Complementarities of FAIR and GDPR in the Context of Longitudinal Studies on Children

Longitudinal studies, which track the trajectories of the same individuals over time, face a unique challenge encapsulated by the phrase "unpredictable long-term future." This concept highlights the tension between designing strategies that ensure FAIR

[1] While we provide recommendations based on literature review and best practices from established cross-national survey projects, this text does not constitute legal advice.

data principles and maintaining GDPR compliance over a span of decades. This challenge is especially relevant for GUIDE, as children's data is initially collected based on the consent provided by the holder of parental responsibility (see Chap. 2 in this book; GDPR Art. 8).

First, a key difficulty in interpreting GDPR concerns obtaining assent from children directly, versus a guardian consenting on their behalf. While minors may agree to participate at a young age, this does not constitute formal consent under the GDPR. National legislation also sets varying age thresholds (e.g., 15 in France, 16 in Germany), after which consent must be obtained directly from minor participants. GUIDE should therefore consider scenarios in which participants reach sufficient maturity to understand the implications of their participation, and exercise their rights, such as accessing, modifying, and deleting their data.

Second, given the longitudinal nature of this design, GUIDE should ensure participants' rights to access or rectify their data in a foreseeable number of years. As data controller, GUIDE should be attentive to the rights and interests of those whose data they hold and adopt proportionate measures to safeguard them. This could be done by defining protocols with the data archive on how a participant could rectify their own data or exercise their other rights. But how would data deletion still be compatible with Open Science? Building the metadata based on controlled vocabularies, such as the Data and Documentation Initiative (Data Documentation Initiative Alliance, 2025), and ensuring this metadata is available in the long run, can be ways to be compliant with FAIR and GDPR, even if an individual exercised their right to be deleted or forgotten. Beyond this example, the technical difficulties of protecting participants' rights should be evaluated, discussed, and solutions should be implemented.

Third, tension rests on the principle of data minimization (GDPR Recital 156) versus unforeseeable future uses of the data. Data minimization means a data controller should limit the collection of personal information to what is directly relevant and necessary to accomplish a specified purpose. Data controllers should only retain the data for as long as necessary given the aforementioned purpose (European Data Protection Supervisor, 2025). Under GDPR, this principle applies to the processing of personal data for archiving purposes in public interest, including scientific or historical research or statistical purposes. In contrast, Open Science emphasizes the benefits that are possible through unforeseeable future uses for data, which creates a tension with the GDPR's objective of protecting individual data privacy. This inherent clash means that GDPR compliance runs contrary to FAIR principles unless long-term procedures are planned, budgeted, tested, and fully implemented (see Chap. 3 in this book). Consequently, FAIR implementation requires long-term planning, especially with regards to the systematic use of protocols and the design and long-term availability of metadata.

Fourth, there is the tension of consent and data usage as GDPR is more restrictive while FAIR is broader in the potential uses of the data. GDPR outlines specific consent, which requires research participants to unambiguously agree to the processing of their data for each specific project they are participating in, and to be informed in advance of the concrete ways in which their data will be used (GDPR

Arts. 6–7, Recital 32). In contrast, Phillips and Knoppers (2019) defined the approach of broad consent for the purposes of certain areas of scientific research in Recital 33. Broad consent allows participants to consent to having their data used in multiple research projects based on a description of broad types of research, only requiring specific consent to certain parts of research projects. Broad consent is used in the case studies described in the next section. There are debates around using consent as the legal basis to fulfill data protection duties when personal data processing is necessary for research. Established practice in social and health research (Phillips & Knoppers, 2019)—for instance, in European infrastructures such as the European Social Survey ERIC (ESS ERIC)—relies on another legal basis, in which processing is being carried out for research purposes in the public interest (GDPR Art. 9(2)(j)). In this scenario, the tasks of data collection and processing are necessary for research and archiving purposes, thus being undertaken in the public interest. For GUIDE, adopting public interest as the legal basis rather than consent would enable data collection in future survey waves, support permanent archiving and long-term data sharing across research fields, and allow use for future, as-yet-unspecified studies.

Lastly, balancing GDPR and FAIR brings operational consequences to digital infrastructures such as GUIDE. For example, data portability (European Data Protection Supervisor, 2025) is simultaneously one of the most demanding rights for organizations to fulfill and one of the least studied in current research. Data portability allows individuals to obtain their data in a "structured, commonly used and machine-readable format" from one data controller to be shared with another data controller (GDPR Art. 20). FAIR's focus on Interoperability frameworks could help enhance data portability by providing technical guidelines and standards. Summing up, resolving the tensions of GDPR and FAIR could mean that even after data collection concludes, GUIDE would need to plan and budget for a long-term infrastructure (see Chap. 10 in this book). Depending on the legal basis used for data processing, this could include revisiting consent and obtaining minors' consent when they reach relevant age thresholds enabling participants' data rights, along with long-term archiving and Findable metadata.

Evaluating Open Science Practices of Four Longitudinal Child-Centered Survey Projects Across Europe

In this section, we examine four case studies of European longitudinal survey projects with child participants. We describe how they operationalize the four FAIR dimensions (Jacobsen et al., 2020; Wilkinson et al., 2016), commenting on aspects that enhance or limit the FAIRness of their data, following the specifications of the FAIR principles laid out by GO FAIR (2025a). Furthermore, we address handling of the GDPR, more specifically how projects handle the topic of *informed consent*, at the core of some of the tensions highlighted above (see Chap. 2 in this book).

Mother and Child Cohort Study (MoBa), Norway

MoBa was brought into existence in the 1990s by a group of perinatal epidemiologists with the aim of detecting causes of serious diseases. Its data also allows researchers to investigate links between health and social variables. MoBa covers children born between 1999 and 2009 and their parents, with a total of more than 114,000 children included in the sample. MoBa collects biodata of mothers, fathers, and children as well as survey data from mothers and fathers during pregnancy and after birth. The study then follows children into youth and adulthood (Magnus et al., 2016; Norwegian Institute of Public Health, 2024).

FAIR

Findability. We found MoBa data to be indexed in health-data specific data catalogues, which is a plus for Findability. Yet, we would recommend indexing it also in catalogues not strictly focused on health, for example in the CESSDA Data Catalogue. This would further improve Findability. A weak point for Findability and Accessibility is that we could not identify the use of DOIs (Digital Object Identifiers) or similar persistent identifiers for any MoBa data. More specifically, we could not find an indication that DOIs are used in the freely available data catalogue entries or data documentation reports (Norwegian Institute of Public Health, 2012).

Accessibility. Regarding access to MoBa data, it should be noted that, in addition to survey data, genomic data and biological material were collected. Hence access is more strictly limited. As emphasized by GO FAIR (2025b) and Wilkinson et al. (2016), Accessibility does not imply unrestricted openness, but rather clear documentation of access procedures and conditions. This information could easily be extracted from the project website which is a plus for MoBa's Accessibility (Norwegian Institute of Public Health, 2023). Namely, researchers can apply for access via the Norwegian Health Data Service (Helsedata, 2025). Access to MoBa data requires a Norwegian electronic ID, meaning international research groups must collaborate with a Norwegian partner. Upon request, MoBa confirmed that the principal investigator must hold doctoral-level research competence and must be affiliated with a Norwegian research institution. Moreover, proposed research questions must align with the purpose of the study and participants' consent, in compliance with the Norwegian Personal Data Act and the GDPR. The MoBa case exemplifies the relevance of GDPR for the Accessibility principle of FAIR.

Interoperability. The MoBa datasets are provided in the common format .SAV which is a plus for Interoperability (Norwegian Mother, Father and Child Cohort Study, 2025a).

Reusability. MoBa is strong on the Reusability principle, providing extensive, and clear data documentation which can be freely downloaded from their website, without registration or similar barriers (Jin, 2016). MoBa strengthens Reusability by maintaining a GitHub repository for sharing syntax, including for variable construction based on its data (Norwegian Mother, Father and Child Cohort Study, 2025b). Yet, a minus for Reusability is the absence of information about license usage.

GDPR

According to the latest study protocol available on the MoBa website (Norwegian Institute of Public Health, 2012), concerning their 2012 study, children are included after consent from the mother, still during the pregnancy. Children are then informed personally about the study at the age of 15. Once they turn 18, MoBa will need informed consent from the youth for the purpose of further storage of their data (Norwegian Institute of Public Health, 2012).

National Educational Panel Study (NEPS), Germany

NEPS aims to track the development of competencies and educational trajectories as well as their conditions and consequences over the entire life span (Leibniz Institute for Educational Trajectories, 2025a). Starting with the first cohort in 2008, it has by now accompanied seven cohorts made up of more than 70,000 participants and about 50,000 parents or educational professionals related to the target child (Leibniz Institute for Educational Trajectories, 2025a).

FAIR

Findability. The availability of DOIs for the datasets enhances the Findability and Accessibility of NEPS data (FDZ-LIfBi, 2024). To further improve Findability, NEPS should be indexed in additional relevant catalogues, such as the GESIS Data Catalogue or the CESSDA Data Catalogue.

Accessibility. Researchers can access NEPS data upon signing a Data Use Agreement with the Leibniz Institute for Educational Trajectories (LIfBi). Researchers need to be affiliated with an institution doing scientific work and provide a description of the research project that the data will be used for (NEPS, 2025a). Datasets containing more sensitive data—for example, more granular geographic information—can be accessed via Remote Desktop Data Access or on-site data security rooms (NEPS, 2025b). The access protocol is clearly described on the project's website which is a plus for NEPS' Accessibility.

Interoperability. The datasets and metadata contained within the datasets are provided in commonly accessible formats, specifically .SAV and .DTA which improves Interoperability (NEPS Network, 2024).

Reusability. NEPS enhances the Reusability of its data by providing clear and extensive data descriptions, viewable directly in the browser via an interactive tool linked on the project website (Leibniz Institute for Educational Trajectories, 2025b) as well as in data documentation such as the survey instrument reports (NEPS, 2013). A strong point for Reusability of NEPS data is that their metadata provided in the freely downloadable documentation is licensed under Creative Commons BY 4.0 (FDZ-LIfBi, 2024).

GDPR

Consent is asked from one parent of participants under age 16. Starting from age 16, participants who remain in the study are asked to consent to one more interview to take place. Consent is not revisited once participants turn 18 (Center for Study Management—Data Protection in Surveys Working Unit, 2023).

Growing Up in Ireland (GUI)

GUI was started in 2006 and aims to inform Irish policymakers in the areas of children, young people and families. So far, data is available for approximately 18,000 children who have been sampled either at 9 months or 9 years of age and followed throughout their life course (Growing Up in Ireland, 2025a). GUI collects survey data from parents, caregivers, teachers, principals, and the children themselves (Growing Up in Ireland, 2025a, 2025b).

FAIR

Findability. All available GUI datafiles have DOIs assigned, which is crucial for enhancing Findability and Accessibility. Findability of GUI data is further improved by the provision of extensive metadata in the Irish Social Science Data Archive catalogue (Irish Social Science Data Archive, 2025). GUI data is also indexed to other relevant data catalogues such as the CESSDA Data Catalogue, further enhancing its Findability.

Accessibility. Researchers can request data access via the Irish Social Science Data Archive. A form containing information about the researchers and the project as well as the signed end user license (signed by the researcher as well as a representative of the institution they are affiliated with) has to be submitted via email to the archive. The access protocol is clearly described on the project website and in its metadata (Irish Social Science Data Archive, 2025); this is a plus for GUI's Accessibility.

Interoperability. Metadata in the Irish Social Science Data Archive employs the CESSDA Vocabulary which enhances its Interoperability. Data is provided in the common format .TAB representing a plus for GUI's Interoperability (Irish Social Science Data Archive, 2025).

Reusability. The Irish Social Science Data Archive catalogue provides extensive and clear descriptions of the data, improving Reusability (Irish Social Science Data Archive, 2025). Copyright lies with the Department of Children, Equality, Disability, Integration, and Youth as explicitly noted in the metadata (Irish Social Science Data Archive, 2025), which is a strength. However, a more common and open license (e.g., Creative Commons) would generally be preferable. It is unclear why such a restrictive license must apply to all materials. For instance, study documentation documents are copyrighted with the condition that "no part of this publication may be reproduced, stored in a retrieval system, or transmitted, in any form or by any means, [...], without the prior permission in writing of the copyright holder" (Williams et al., 2019), which seems unnecessarily restrictive.

GDPR

Parental consent of one parent is required for participants under 18 years of age. We have not found evidence that consent would be revisited once participants turn 18. In the case that a parent was under age 16, both the underage parent and one of their parents or guardians would need to provide consent. Parents being 16 years and older can provide consent for them and their child to participate in the study.

ELFE: French Longitudinal Study of Children

The ELFE study launched in 2011 and followed more than 18,000 children from birth to adulthood, with a primary focus on health while accounting for social and environmental context factors (Charles et al., 2020; INED, 2025a). The majority of ELFE's survey data stems from parents. Yet, skills tests and biological measures are taken from children as well as some survey data (INED, 2025a).

FAIR

Findability. ELFE makes scarce use of DOIs or similar persistent identifiers. Currently, only a few datasets have been assigned DOIs (T. Siméon, personal communication, January 7, 2025). This severely limits ELFE's Findability and Accessibility. However, ELFE's Findability is enhanced by the fact that the study is indexed in data catalogues. It is, for example, listed in the catalogue of France Cohortes (France Cohortes, 2025), a portal focused on French cohort studies (France Cohortes, 2025) as well as in the MOLGENIS data catalogue (MOLGENIS, 2025a; Swertz et al., 2010, 2022; van der Velde et al., 2019). The latter is a research data platform, including a data catalogue, specifically for health data. It also offers other features facilitating research collaboration (for further information, see MOLGENIS [2025b]). We would recommend furthermore indexing ELFE data in catalogues not strictly focused on health, for example the CESSDA Data Catalogue, to enhance Findability.

Accessibility. The data access protocol is clearly outlined on the project's website (INED, 2025b), although no specification of it was found in the metadata, we had access to. Access requires initial registration, followed by submission of a request to the ELFE Data Access Committee (Comité d'accès aux données, CADE), which determines whether access is granted. Prospective users must then sign a user agreement, after which the dataset is provided. The entire process typically takes between one and two months (T. Siméon, personal communication, January 7, 2025).

Interoperability. The ELFE datasets and metadata contained within the datasets are provided in the common formats .CSV and .SAS which is a plus for Interoperability (INED, 2025c).

Reusability. In general, the data are extensively and clearly described. A limitation, however, is that some documentation is, to date, available only in French. Reusability would also be strengthened by the clear provision of a license for the data and metadata.

GDPR

Consent for study participation is asked from both parents or from the mother alone, with the father being informed of his right to deny consent for participation (Charles et al., 2020). This holds for children up to age 14. From age 15 to 18, both parental and child consent is requested. Consent is not revisited once participants turn 18 (T. Siméon, personal communication, January 7, 2025). Furthermore, underage parents or parents who were not capable of giving informed consent were excluded from the study (INED, 2025a).

Good Practice Case: SHARE ERIC

In Table 8.1, column 1 describes SHARE ERIC's good practices, column 2 classifies practices by GDPR and FAIR, and column 3 zooms into the FAIR principles where applicable. As a European-wide, longitudinal research infrastructure, many of these good practices should be reflected upon and adapted to GUIDE's focus on children.

Recommendations for GUIDE's Approach to Open Science

Given the good practices and case studies above, we propose a timeline of recommendations for GUIDE assuming a 24-month lead to launch date, which might be adapted by other projects considering such approaches.

Table 8.1 Good practice case: SHARE ERIC

Good practice SHARE ERIC	Classification FAIR/ GDPR	Subclassification FAIR
Data anonymized, attempts at re-identification prohibited as per data user agreement	GDPR	
Data freely accessible with only condition being exclusively scientific usage Safeguarded by requiring (quick & easy!) registration, asking prospective users to indicate affiliation to academic/ scientific institution & info about planned scientific use	Accessibility	**A1**. Data and metadata are retrievable by their identifier using a standardized communications protocol **A1.1** The protocol is open, free, and universally implementable **A1.2** The protocol allows for an authentication and authorization procedure, where necessary
Documentation freely available (without registration as user): – Guides to SHARE ERIC database – Methodology & compliance profiles – All questionnaires – Scales manual – Information on cross-wave comparisons – Data management plan – Metadata freely available to browse in special tool (https://www.share-datadocutool.org/)	Findability, Reusability, Interoperability	**F2**. Data are described with rich metadata **F4**. Data and metadata are registered or indexed in a searchable resource **R1**. Data and metadata are richly described with a plurality of accurate and relevant attributes **I1**. Data and metadata use formal, accessible, shared, and broadly applicable language for knowledge representation **I2**. Data and metadata use vocabularies that follow FAIR principles
Datasets provided in common formats (.dta, .sav) which can be used with free statistical software such as R	Interoperability, Reusability	**I1**. Data and metadata use formal, accessible, shared, and broadly applicable language for knowledge representation **R1.3**. Data and metadata meet domain-relevant community standards
Datasets made available to users in timely manner (i.e., promptly after data collection)	Reusability	**R1.3**. Data and metadata meet domain-relevant community standards
Instruction of correct citation of data provided, as well as request to inform SHARE ERIC central team about publications	Findability, Reusability	**R1**. Data and metadata are richly described with a plurality of accurate and relevant attributes **F4**. Data and metadata are registered or indexed in a searchable resource

(continued)

Table 8.1 (continued)

Good practice SHARE ERIC	Classification FAIR/GDPR	Subclassification FAIR
Provides information on data linking, e.g., linking SHARE ERIC data with administrative records from different countries	Interoperability	**I1**. Data and metadata use formal, accessible, shared, and broadly applicable language for knowledge representation **I2**. Data and metadata use vocabularies that follow FAIR principles **I3**. Data and metadata include qualified references to other data and metadata
DOI prefix and suffix allow easy identification of specific wave of SHARE ERIC	Findability	**F1**. Data and metadata are assigned to a globally unique and persistent identifier
Member of FAIRsharing initiative (https://fairsharing.org)	Findability, Interoperability	**F4**. Data and metadata are registered or indexed in a searchable resource **I3**. Data and metadata include qualified references to other data and metadata
Data-reuse promoted by provision of generated modules (e.g., imputations, weights, ISCED-codes) as well as a teaching dataset (easySHARE) for training of inexperienced users	Reusability	**R1.2**. Data and metadata are associated with detailed provenance **R1.3**. Data and metadata meet domain-relevant community standards

Months 1–6

- Training of team members in FAIR and GDPR frameworks using materials of SSHOC initiative (see Chap. 3 in this book; SSHOC, 2025).

Months 7–12

- Look into becoming a member of FAIRsharing initiative (https://fairsharing.org).
- Appoint a Data Protection Officer (DPO), identify data controller and data processors, and sign data protection agreements with the data processors.
- Design the data workflow from data reception to data dissemination, including domain-relevant metadata to be selected using controlled vocabularies (Maineri, 2022), informed by best practices (e.g., CESSDA Vocabulary see FAIR-sharing.org, 2026; Data Documentation Initiative Alliance, 2025; Saldanha Bach Estevao & Klas, 2024), and shared on the project's website. Metadata should

remain accessible even if datasets are no longer available and should be assigned DOIs and licensed under Creative Commons.

- Once a controlled vocabulary has been chosen, plan and budget for a timely consultation of substantive experts from relevant disciplines to provide input on relevant metadata contents (i.e., keywords, topic classification, kind of data, time method, mode of data collection and type of research instrument) to enhance Findability.
- Consult the FAIR Implementation Profile, a 21-item checklist (Schultes et al., 2020) and the European Publications Office on metadata quality criteria (Publications Office of the European Union, 2025).
- Design the archive system architecture using resources such as Agasøster et al. (2022) to ensure Interoperability of the data and metadata. Providing data and metadata in commonly used and machine-readable formats. Consider data security measures (e.g., encryption, access controls, regular data backups).

Month 13–18

- Prepare the source materials and translations that will be shared with respondents (e.g., privacy notices/policies, legal basis for data processing, their rights, data access protocol; see Chap. 2 in this book) that includes reference to a data breach response plan, including clear protocols for detecting, notifying, containing, and mitigating data breaches.

Months 19–24

- Establish regular communication between the DPO, central team, and national teams on data protection policies and operations, data processing activities, and monitor compliance with data protection laws.
- Publish GUIDE's data management plan documenting FAIRness (e.g., SHARE ERIC, 2023).

During Data Collection

- Publish the data access protocol on the project website and in the metadata (e.g., Shibboleth, 2025).
- Design an interactive browser-based tool about each variable shared on the project website (e.g., ESS ERIC: European Social Survey ERIC, 2025; NEPS: Leibniz Institute for Educational Trajectories, 2025b; SHARE ERIC: Centerdata, 2025).

- Index the project in relevant data catalogues (e.g., CESSDA Data Catalogue, MOLGENIS, ODISSEI Portal, re3data.org Registry of Research Data Repositories).
- Set up a public repository (e.g., GitHub, OSF) where researchers share analysis code to enhance Reusability.

After Data Collection

- Publish the Creative Commons license along with DOIs for all datasets, similar to metadata.
- Actively promote data reuse. For example, SHARE ERIC provides generated modules—such as imputations, weights and ISCED-codes—and a teaching dataset (easySHARE) for training and inexperienced users (SHARE ERIC, 2024).

Future Directions

Balancing the FAIRness of GUIDE's data with the requirements of GDPR remains a critical, ongoing topic. Since FAIRness is a spectrum, the degree of compliance achieved will likely evolve as technologies and data practices advance. While data confidentiality and security during access to researchers were priorities in all studied cases, the implementation of FAIR in longitudinal studies with children varied. GUIDE and other longitudinal studies with children could develop a FAIR and data protection code of conduct, similar to developments in health research (Litton, 2017).

FAIR and GDPR are highly technical concepts, combining computer science and legal terminology. Scientists conducting research on children are not necessarily familiar with these concepts. As seen in this chapter, FAIR applies not only to the storage of datasets, but also to analytical workflows, which need to be categorized, described, and stored in a way that supports their Findability and Reusability. FAIR data depends heavily on how it is stored, registered, indexed, and preserved. GUIDE should consider that data protection and FAIR require an array of knowledge, skills and competencies, which require training and long-term planning to achieve. In this context, the chapter provides a detailed list of recommendations for the pilot and initial GUIDE Wave. Rooted in FAIR and GDPR, practices should be revisited continuously to ensure GUIDE meets the highest standards in Open Science and data protection.

References

Agasøster, B., Bergseth, G. H., Beuster, B., Bidargaddi, A., Risnes, Ø., Skjåk, K. K., Stavestrand, E. (2022). *D5.13 Recommendations for a FAIR compliant integrated data and metadata repository (ESS as a service)*. Zenodo. https://doi.org/10.5281/zenodo.6564151

Centerdata. (2025). *SHARE data & documentation tool*. https://www.share-datadocutool.org/

Charles, M. A., Thierry, X., Lanoe, J.-L., Bois, C., Dufourg, M.-N., Popa, R., Cheminat, M., Zaros, C., & Geay, B. (2020). Cohort Profile: The French national cohort of children (ELFE): Birth to 5 years. *International Journal of Epidemiology, 49*(2), 368–369j. https://doi.org/10.1093/ije/dyz227

Data Documentation Initiative Alliance. (2025). *Supporting data producers and data consumers*. https://ddialliance.org/

European Social Survey ERIC. (2025). *ESS Data Portal—Variable viewer—ESS11 integrated file, edition 2.0*. https://ess.sikt.no/en/datafile/242aaa39-3bbb-40f5-98bf-bfb1ce53d8ef?tab=1

FAIRsharing.org. (2026). *CESSDA VS; CESSDA Vocabulary Service*. Retrieved June 26, 2026, from https://doi.org/10.25504/FAIRsharing.5c7cec

FDZ-LIfBi. (2024). *Data manual NEPS Starting Cohort 1—Newborns, education from the very beginning, scientific use file version 11.0.0*. Leibniz Institute for Educational Trajectories, National Educational Panel Study. https://www.neps-data.de/Data-Center/Data-and-Documentation/Start-Cohort-Newborns/105157-NEPSSC11100

France Cohortes. (2025). *ELFE—French Longitudinal Study from Childhood*. https://francecohortes.org/en/cohorts/cohorts-directory/ELFE

GO FAIR. (2025a). *FAIR principles*. https://www.go-fair.org/fair-principles/

GO FAIR. (2025b). *A1.2: The protocol allows for an authentication and authorisation procedure where necessary*. https://www.go-fair.org/fair-principles/a1-2-protocol-allows-authentication-authorisation-required/

Growing Up in Ireland. (2025a). *Growing up in Ireland*. https://www.growingup.gov.ie/

Growing Up in Ireland. (2025b). *About growing up in Ireland*. https://www.growingup.gov.ie/about-growing-up-in-ireland/

Helsedata. (2025). *The Norwegian Mother, Father and Child Cohort Study (MoBa)*. https://helsedata.no/en/forvaltere/norwegian-institute-of-public-health/norwegian-mother-father-and-child-cohort-study-moba/

INED. (2025a). *The ELFE study—Background to the study*. https://www.elfe-france.fr/en/the-elfe-study/background-to-the-study/

INED. (2025b). *ELFE—Access to data & questionnaires*. https://www.elfe-france.fr/en/the-research/access-to-data-and-questionnaires/

INED. (2025c). *Étude longitudinale française depuis l'enfance* [Database]. https://doi.org/10.48756/ined-inserm-elfe-8642

European Commission. (2024). *Open science*. European Research Executive Agency. https://rea.ec.europa.eu/open-science_en

European Commission, Directorate-General for Research and Innovation. (2019). *Future of scholarly publishing and scholarly communication: Report of the Expert Group to the European Commission*. Publications Office of the European Union. https://doi.org/10.2777/836532

European Commission, Directorate-General for Research and Innovation. (2021). *Horizon Europe, open science—Early knowledge and data sharing, and open collaboration*. Publications Office of the European Union. https://doi.org/10.2777/18252

European Data Protection Supervisor. (2025). *Data minimisation*. European Data Protection Supervisor. https://www.edps.europa.eu/data-protection/data-protection/glossary/d_en

Irish Social Science Data Archive. (2025). *Growing Up in Ireland (GUI) Cohort '98 (Child Cohort) Wave 5—25 years, 2023*. https://doi.org/10.7929/ISSDA/7IANG6

Jacobsen, A., de Miranda Azevedo, R., Juty, N., Batista, D., Coles, S., Cornet, R., Courtot, M., Crosas, M., Dumontier, M., Evelo, C. T., Goble, C., Guizzardi, G., Hansen, K. K., Hasnain, A., Hettne, K., Heringa, J., Hooft, R. W. W., Imming, M., Jeffery, K. G., ... Schultes, E. (2020).

FAIR principles: Interpretations and implementation considerations. *Data Intelligence, 2*(1–2), 10–29. https://doi.org/10.1162/dint_r_00024

Jin, F. (2016). *Questions documentation: Questionnaire 1, 15th week of gestation: The Norwegian Mother and Child Cohort Study (MoBa).* Norwegian Institute of Public Health. https://www.fhi.no/en/ch/studies/moba/for-forskere-artikler/questionnaires-from-moba/

Leibniz Institute for Educational Trajectories. (2025a). *National Education Panel Study NEPS.* https://www.lifbi.de/en-us/Start/Research/Large-Scale-Projects/NEPS-National-Educational-Panel-Study

Leibniz Institute for Educational Trajectories. (2025b). *Variable search.* https://variablesearch.lifbi.de/

Litton, J.-E. (2017). We must urgently clarify data-sharing rules. *Nature, 541*(7638), 437. https://doi.org/10.1038/541437a

Magnus, P., Birke, C., Vejrup, K., Haugan, A., Alsaker, E., Daltveit, A. K., & Stoltenberg, C. (2016). Cohort profile update: The Norwegian Mother and Child Cohort Study (MoBa). *International Journal of Epidemiology, 45*(2), 382–388. https://doi.org/10.1093/ije/dyw029

Maineri, A. M. (2022). *Controlled vocabularies for the social sciences: What they are, and why we need them.* Zenodo.

MOLGENIS. (2025a). *ELFE Étude longitudinale française depuis l'enfance (French longitudinal study of children).* https://molgeniscatalogue.org/all/collections/ELFE

MOLGENIS. (2025b). *For scientific data.* https://molgenis.org/

NEPS. (2013). *Startkohorte 3: Klasse 5 (SC3)—Welle 1 Erhebungsinstrumente (Feldversion).* Universität Bamberg, Nationales Bildungspanel. https://www.neps-data.de/Portals/0/NEPS/Datenzentrum/Forschungsdaten/SC3/1-0-0/SC3_Q_w1.pdf

NEPS. (2025a). *Data use agreements.* https://www.neps-data.de/Data-Center/Data-Access/Data-Use-Agreements

NEPS. (2025b). *Access to NEPS data.* https://www.neps-data.de/Data-Center/Data-Access

NEPS Network. (2024). *National Educational Panel Study, scientific use file of Starting Cohort Newborns.* Leibniz Institute for Educational Trajectories. https://doi.org/10.5157/NEPS:SC1:11.0.0

Norwegian Institute of Public Health. (2012). *Norwegian Mother and Child Cohort Study revised protocol end of enrollment—Protocol II* (Tech. Rep.). https://www.fhi.no/globalassets/dokumenterfiler/studier/den-norske-mor-far-og-barn--undersokelsenmoba/protokoll/2012-moba-protokoll.pdf

Norwegian Institute of Public Health. (2023). *Access to data and biological material from the Norwegian Mother, Father and Child Cohort Study (MoBa).* https://www.fhi.no/en/ch/studies/moba/for-forskere-artikler/research-and-data-access

Norwegian Institute of Public Health. (2024). *Questionnaires from MoBa.* https://www.fhi.no/en/ch/studies/moba/for-forskere-artikler/questionnaires-from-moba/#19-years-questionnaire

Norwegian Mother, Father and Child Cohort Study. (2025a). *MoBa "variable list" and "biological material form"—Data from the Norwegian Mother, Father and Child Cohort variable list.* https://www.fhi.no/en/publ/forms/Form-for-request-for-data-and-bio-in-MoBa/

Norwegian Mother, Father and Child Cohort Study. (2025b). *Welcome to MoBa Wiki.* https://github.com/folkehelseinstituttet/Fhi.MoBa/wiki

Phillips, M., & Knoppers, B. M. (2019). Whose commons? Data protection as a legal limit of open science. *Journal of Law, Medicine and Ethics, 47*(1), 106–111. https://doi.org/10.1177/1073110519840489

Publications Office of the European Union. (2025). *Metadata quality assessment methodology.* https://data.europa.eu/mqa/methodology?locale=en

Saldanha Bach Estevao, J., & Klas, C.-P. (2024). Enhancing FAIR compliance: A controlled vocabulary for mapping Social Sciences survey variables. *IASSIST Quarterly, 48*(2). https://doi.org/10.29173/iq1118

SHARE ERIC. (2023). *Survey of Health, Ageing and Retirement in Europe (SHARE) data management plan.* https://share-eric.eu/fileadmin/user_upload/Other_Publications/Data_Management_Plan.pdf

SHARE ERIC. (2024). *easySHARE* (Release version 9.0.0). SHARE-ERIC. https://doi.org/10.6103/SHARE.easy.900

Schultes, E., Magagna, B., Hettne, K. M., Pergl, R., Suchanek, M., & Kuhn, T. (2020). Reusable FAIR implementation profiles as accelerators of FAIR convergence. In G. Grossmann & S. Ram (Eds.), *Advances in conceptual modeling* (pp. 138–147). Springer International Publishing.

Shibboleth. (2025). *The Shibboleth Project.* https://www.shibboleth.net/about-us/the-shibboleth-project/

SSHOC. (2025). *Training—SSHOPENCLOUD.* https://sshopencloud.eu/training

Swertz, M., van Enckevort, E., Oliveira, J. L., Fortier, I., Bergeron, J., Thurin, N. H., Hyde, E., Kellmann, A., Pahoueshnja, R., Sturkenboom, M., Cunnington, M., Nybo Andersen, A.-M., Marcon, Y., Gonçalves, G., & Gini, R. (2022). Towards an interoperable ecosystem of research cohort and real-world data catalogues enabling multi-center studies. *Yearbook of Medical Informatics, 31*(1), 262–272. https://doi.org/10.1055/s-0042-1742522

Swertz, M. A., Dijkstra, M., Adamusiak, T., van der Velde, J. K., Kanterakis, A., Roos, E. T., Lops, J., Thorisson, G. A., Arends, D., Byelas, G., Muilu, J., Brookes, A. J., de Brock, E. O., Jansen, R. C., & Parkinson, H. (2010). The MOLGENIS toolkit: Rapid prototyping of biosoftware at the push of a button. *BMC Bioinformatics, 11*(Suppl. 12), Article S12. https://doi.org/10.1186/1471-2105-11-S12-S12

Ursin, G., & Bentzen, H. B. (2021). Open science and sharing personal data widely—Legally impossible for Europeans? *Acta Oncologica, 60*(12), 1555–1556. https://doi.org/10.1080/0284186X.2021.1995894

van der Velde, K. J., Imhann, F., Charbon, B., Pang, C., van Enckevort, D., Slofstra, M., Barbieri, R., Alberts, R., Hendriksen, D., Kelpin, F., de Haan, M., de Boer, T., Haakma, S., Stroomberg, C., Scholtens, S., van de Geijn, G.-J., Festen, E. A. M., Weersma, R. K., & Swertz, M. A. (2019). MOLGENIS research: Advanced bioinformatics data software for non-bioinformaticians. *Bioinformatics, 35*(6), 1076–1078. https://doi.org/10.1093/bioinformatics/bty742

Vicente-Saez, R., & Martínez-Fuentes, C. (2018). Open science now: A systematic literature review for an integrated definition. *Journal of Business Research, 88*, 428–436. https://doi.org/10.1016/j.jbusres.2017.12.043

Wilkinson, M. D., Dumontier, M., Aalbersberg, I. J. J., Appleton, G., Axton, M., Baak, A., Blomberg, N., Boiten, J. W., da Silva Santos, L. B., Bourne, P. E., Bouwman, J., Brookes, A. J., Clark, T., Crosas, M., Dillo, I., Dumon, O., Edmunds, S., Evelo, C. T., Finkers, R., ... Mons, B. (2016). The FAIR guiding principles for scientific data management and stewardship. *Scientific Data, 3*(1), Article 160018. https://doi.org/10.1038/sdata.2016.18

Williams, J., Murray, A., O'Mahony, D., Quail, A., O'Reilly, C., Thornton, M., & Neary, M. (2019). *Growing Up in Ireland: The pilot phase of the Child Cohort at 17/18 years of age and recommendations* (Technical Series No. 2019-7). ESRI/TCD/DCYA. https://www.growingup.gov.ie/pubs/20190715-Cohort-98-at-17-pilot-report-2019-7.pdf

Diana Zavala-Rojas (Ph.D.) is a social scientist interested in all aspects of the human data lifecycle. She is a specialist in multinational, multiregional and multilingual comparative surveys. She is the Deputy Director of RECSM and a member of the Core Scientific Team (CST) of the European Social Survey (ESS).

Hannah Schwarz (M.Sc) is a senior research manager at Research and Expertise Centre for Survey Methodology (RECSM). Her research focuses on survey response quality. She holds a master's in social science research from the University of Amsterdam and has previously worked for the Comparative Study of Electoral Systems (CSES) at GESIS – Leibniz Institute for the Social Sciences.

Chapter 9
Best Practices for Data Harmonization and Comparability of Child Wellbeing Across Europe

Sabine Düval, Susanne Kuger, and Lynda M. Sagrestano

Ensuring Cross-National Comparability: Best Practices in Data Harmonization

Ensuring cross-national comparability is a core methodological requirement in cross-national research on child wellbeing, especially in large-scale, longitudinal studies. Without strong comparability, findings cannot be meaningfully interpreted across different cultural and national contexts (van de Vijver et al., 2019). When measures lack comparability, it is unclear whether observed differences among countries reflect true variation in child wellbeing or are merely artifacts of biased measurement instruments and procedures. Such bias can undermine the validity of cross-national comparisons on multiple levels. Differences in the understanding of constructs, cultural relevance of items, or survey administration can all affect how questions are interpreted and answered across countries (van de Vijver & Leung, 1997). When indicators are biased, the meaning of responses differs across contexts, reducing the utility of the data for comparative research (van de Vijver et al., 2019). Addressing these risks requires careful *ex-ante* design of instruments and procedures and *ex-post* analytical checks. Measurement invariance testing has emerged as a central tool to empirically evaluate whether constructs function equivalently across countries and over time (Jude & Kuger, 2018).

Testing for measurement invariance is particularly relevant when self-report survey data are used to capture key constructs, as is frequently the case in child

S. Düval (✉) · S. Kuger · L. M. Sagrestano
German Youth Institute, Munich, Germany
e-mail: dueval@dji.de

S. Düval
Federal Institute for Population Research, Wiesbaden, Germany

S. Kuger
LMU Munich, Munich, Germany

L. K. Taylor et al. (eds.), *Growing Up in Digital Europe*, Springer Series on Child and Family Studies, https://doi.org/10.1007/978-3-032-30592-3_9

wellbeing research. Unlike more structured or externally validated methods—such as standardized achievement tests, behavioral observations, or physiological indicators—self-reports rely on respondents' subjective interpretation of item wording and response formats. This makes them more susceptible to cultural and linguistic variation in how questions are understood and answered, increasing the likelihood of measurement bias across groups. Establishing measurement invariance is therefore essential to ensure that observed differences in self-reported outcomes reflect true variation in the construct of interest rather than systematic discrepancies in interpretation.

If a construct lacks invariance—or is *variant*—it suggests that the underlying concept is not interpreted or responded to in the same way across cultural contexts. As a result, cross-national comparisons of mean levels, structural relations, or longitudinal trends may be misleading, because observed differences might stem from measurement artifacts rather than substantive phenomena. This has direct implications for cross-national studies, such as Growing Up in Digital Europe (GUIDE), which rely on questionnaire items to measure central outcomes such as wellbeing and digital media use. Large-scale studies such as PISA (e.g., problem-solving tasks) or TIMSS (e.g., mathematics and science assessments) assess their primary outcomes through standardized performance-based instruments measured through direct measures such as scaled competence tests. GUIDE, by comparison, captures its main constructs solely through self-reported perceptions and behaviors, which makes the data more vulnerable to bias and increases the importance of ensuring measurement validity and comparability across countries.

Ensuring cross-national comparability has been a central concern in the development of GUIDE. As the first cross-nationally comparable, nationally representative longitudinal study of child and youth wellbeing in Europe, GUIDE builds on extensive groundwork laid in its predecessor projects, COORDINATE and GUIDEPREP (see Chap. 1 in this book). These earlier phases focused on refining the conceptual and methodological foundations of cross-national comparability. Key efforts included aligning indicators across existing studies, developing a harmonized questionnaire (see Chap. 5 in this book), developing rigorous translation and cultural adaptation protocols, coordinating a common sampling framework (see Chap. 4 in this book), standardizing survey administration, and conducting a multi-country pilot to test functional comparability.

This chapter builds on these preparatory steps and offers practical guidance for the design and implementation of harmonized cross-national studies. It outlines the main challenges to comparability, such as construct, method, and item bias. It also presents methodological strategies to improve validity and reliability, drawing on GUIDE's design as a best-practice model. Finally, it addresses the issue of comparability after data collection, with a focus on measurement invariance testing. Using 2019 TIMSS data from France, Germany, and Norway, the chapter illustrates how to test for invariance across countries through multi-group confirmatory factor analysis.

Key Challenges of Cross-National Comparability

In large-scale cross-national longitudinal studies such as GUIDE, differences in cultural context, language, and response styles can lead to variation in how questions are interpreted and answered, even when the same instruments are used across countries and waves (Johnson & van de Vijver, 2003). Three core threats to comparability are commonly distinguished: construct bias, method bias, and item bias (van de Vijver & Leung, 1997; van de Vijver et al., 2019). At the heart of these concerns lies the concept of measurement invariance, which refers to the requirement that a given construct carries the same meaning across countries and time points (Desa et al., 2018; Rutkowski & Svetina, 2014). Without sufficient measurement invariance, observed differences may reflect measurement artifacts rather than true differences in the underlying constructs. The following section outlines three major types of bias that pose risks to cross-national comparability (for a short overview, see Table 9.1).

Table 9.1 Key types of bias affecting cross-national comparability in survey research

Type of bias	Definition	Examples
Construct bias	• The construct does not carry the same meaning across cultures • Definitions may only partially overlap • Certain aspects may be underrepresented or culturally irrelevant	• "Happiness": linked to personal success in individualistic cultures vs. social harmony in collectivist cultures • "Digital media use": focus on desktops vs. smartphones depending on country context
Method bias	• Bias introduced through methodological difference • Arises from sampling procedures, survey administration, or mode of data collection • Can distort observed differences between groups	• Sampling: school-based vs. population registries • Mode: interviewer-led (more social desirability bias) vs. self-administered
Item bias	• Respondents with the same underlying trait respond differently to the same item • Caused by poor translation, ambiguous wording, or cultural mismatch • Items may evoke unintended meanings	• "Family": interpreted as nuclear in some cultures, extended in others • "Leisure": includes home-based vs. outdoor activities depending on climate • Idioms or culturally specific terms misinterpreted

Note This table summarizes the three major types of bias that threaten the comparability of cross-national survey data (van de Vijver & Leung, 1997; van de Vijver et al., 2019)

Construct Bias

Construct bias arises when the understanding of a construct differs across countries or cultures. This can occur when definitions of the construct only partially overlap between cultures, or not all aspects of the construct relevant for each culture are measured. Further sources of construct bias include content that is inappropriate, and poor selection of items in overly short instruments leading to inadequate representation of the construct (van de Vijver & Poortinga, 1997). For example, conceptualizations of "child wellbeing" can vary in culturally specific ways, affecting what is measured and how it is interpreted. In individualistic cultures, wellbeing is viewed more as a personal characteristic linked to independence and achievement, whereas in collectivistic cultures, it is associated with social embeddedness and belonging (Exenberger et al., 2019). As a result, measures developed in individualistic and collectivist cultures may include different indicators that reflect the different cultural contexts (Kitayama et al., 2000). For example, in individualistic cultures, happiness is derived from personal achievement, which in turn confers personal worth. In contrast, in collectivist cultures, happiness is derived from social relationships leading to interdependence, social harmony, and mutual understanding (Kitayama & Markus, 2000; Kitayama et al., 2007; Uchida et al., 2004).

Method Bias

Method bias refers to systematic distortions that arise from differences in the methodological setup of comparative empirical studies. Such biases can compromise the comparability of findings and may lead to erroneous interpretations of observed differences among study populations. In fact, method bias tends to have a globally upward or downward influence on cross-cultural score differences, meaning it will become part of global mean differences, making it hard to be factored out, and can be easily mistaken for real differences (van de Vijver, 2018). These distortions can originate in the sampling (i.e., sampling bias), structural characteristics of the instrument (i.e., instrument bias), or administration (i.e., administration bias). Sampling bias results from incompatibility of samples due to cross-cultural variation of sample characteristics that have a bearing on the target measures (He & van de Vijver, 2012). This bias may stem from the use of different sampling techniques (e.g., strict random probability versus non-probability sampling), differences in how the target population is defined (e.g., if children's age ranges differ or if some countries oversample vulnerable groups), or if different sampling frames are used (e.g., population registries versus recruiting children through schools[1]), leading to coverage errors (van de Vijver et al., 2019).

[1] This systematically excludes children who do not attend school, for example, due to medical conditions or homeschooling.

Instrument bias occurs when specific characteristics of a measurement instrument systematically distort respondents' answers. One common source of such bias is culturally influenced response styles, particularly in personality and attitude inventories (van de Vijver et al., 2019). These response styles represent systematic patterns, including acquiescence, which is the tendency to agree with items regardless of their content; midpoint responding, the inclination to choose neutral or moderate options irrespective of item meaning; extreme responding, favoring the endpoints of a scale regardless of item content; and social desirability, answering in ways perceived as socially acceptable or favorable (van de Vijver & Leung, 1997). Cross-cultural differences in these response tendencies are often linked to background characteristics such as socioeconomic status and education level and are more commonly observed among individuals from collectivistic cultures (Harzing, 2006; Smith & Fischer, 2008). These biases can significantly affect scores on target constructs such as child wellbeing.

Administration bias refers to differences in the administration conditions of the survey, including data collection modes, (ambiguous) instructions, interaction between administrator and respondents (e.g., halo effects), and communication problems (e.g., language differences, taboo topic) (He & van de Vijver, 2012). For example, interviewer-administered surveys are more susceptible to social desirability effects than self-administered surveys (Rickwood & Coleman-Rose, 2023). Visibility bias may occur due to variations in whether participants can see upcoming items based on the device used. Ambiguous instructions, literacy issues, and social dynamics in the interview situation may also introduce method bias (van de Vijver, 2018).

Item Bias

Item bias occurs when the same item is interpreted differently in different countries or cultural contexts, such that individuals with the same underlying level of the construct respond differently to that item (van de Vijver et al., 2019). This bias typically arises from linguistic and cultural factors, such as poor translation, culturally specific terms, inadequate or complex item formulation (e.g., use of double negatives), items invoking more than one trait or characteristic, and cultural differences in the relevance or appropriateness of the item content (Davidov et al., 2014; van de Vijver & Poortinga, 1997). For example, one study examining item bias in the quality-of-life scales found that items referring to family were interpreted differently, with the Dutch sample considering the nuclear family and the Spanish participants considering extended family, in part due to terminology choices in translation (Benítez et al., 2022).

Strategies to Address Challenges of Cross-National Comparability

Minimizing bias in cross-cultural research typically involves a combination of strategies that span the entire research process, from study design to implementation to data analysis (He & van de Vijver, 2012), and which are applied in two key stages. The first stage focuses on the period *prior to data collection*, emphasizing the development of standardized measurement constructs, harmonized instruments, and unified sampling procedures. The second stage targets *post-data collection* comparability through analytical validation techniques. The following section presents both stages in detail, outlining the specific procedures used to promote and assess comparability before and after data collection.

Maximizing Comparability Prior to Data Collection

Several steps can be taken prior to data collection to reduce bias and enhance cross-national comparability. At the conceptual level, this involves carefully defining and harmonizing measurement constructs to ensure they are relevant and meaningful across cultural contexts. For example, the construct of digital media use today encompasses a wide range of activities and devices that have evolved over time and may vary in relevance across cultures. A clear and consistent delineation of the construct is necessary to ensure that all participating countries measure the same phenomenon and avoid construct bias (van de Vijver et al., 2019).

Theoretical constructs must then be operationalized through concrete, measurable indicators that reflect current and country-specific realities. Whereas earlier surveys measured digital media use solely by assessing desktop computer use, children today live in digitally rich home environments with regular access to smartphones and tablets (e.g., Konca, 2022). Therefore, adapting existing or developing new indicators that capture contemporary media landscapes and diverse usage patterns across countries is necessary (van de Vijver et al., 2019). To minimize bias, researchers can apply strategies such as decentering (i.e., developing instruments simultaneously in multiple cultures and retaining only those items that function equivalently across contexts) and convergence (i.e., identifying shared elements within independently developed instruments from different cultural settings). Combining items across measures that represent both the overlaps and the diversity of constructs leads to a more comprehensive picture of the construct across cultures (He & van de Vijver, 2012).

Alternatively, bias can be reduced through carefully choosing measures for adoption (i.e., close translation to the target language), adaption (i.e., translation with cultural modification), or assembly (i.e., selecting items from multiple instruments to create a more suitable measure; He & van de Vijver, 2012). The translation of questionnaires to ensure comparability between countries is a key issue in cross-country surveys (Eremenco et al., 2005; Korsnakova & Dept, 2020; Zavala-Rojas et al., 2022). Moreover, children's responses may be especially affected by the style and wording of the questions (Krähenbühl & Blades, 2006).

Cognitive interviewing is a qualitative method used in survey design and evaluation to assess how items are functioning (see Chap. 5 in this book). It involves asking individuals to share their interpretation of items, thereby providing insight into cognitive processes underlying item interpretation (Boeije & Willis, 2013). Cognitive probes, used after each item or at the end of the survey, can uncover problems with wording and terminology, as well as what the items capture more broadly (Willis, 2005). Cognitive interview data is then analyzed and used to adjust and harmonize items. In the cross-national context, cognitive interviewing can be used to identify and remediate issues stemming from construct, method, and item bias (Fitzgerald et al., 2009).

Finally, careful attention must be given to the design and administration of the survey. Standardizing the questionnaire format, including question order, response scales, and instructions, ensures that all respondents receive the same stimuli, minimizing administration differences. Sampling procedures should be harmonized across countries, employing strict random sampling strategies and clear inclusion criteria to ensure that samples are comparable (see Chap. 4 in this book; van de Vijver et al., 2019). Fieldwork protocols should be standardized, including interviewer training, data collection mode (e.g., digital vs. paper), and informed consent and data privacy procedures (see Chaps. 2 and 3 in this book). Consistency reduces the risk that differences in data collection methods bias the results, thereby supporting valid cross-national comparisons.

GUIDE's Approach to Cross-National Comparability

GUIDE was conceived and designed as a harmonized, pan-European longitudinal study (see Chap. 1 in this book). It aims to ensure cross-national comparability and reduce bias in the measurement of child wellbeing across participating countries. GUIDE is structured to ensure that observed differences among countries reflect true variation in child wellbeing rather than methodological artifacts. The foundation for this objective was supported by two preparatory projects, COORDINATE (Horizon 2020, Grant Agreement No. 101008589) and GUIDEPREP (Horizon Europe, Grant Agreement No. 101078945), which focused on developing and testing the key components of the survey design (e.g., instrument development, translation procedures, sampling strategies, and fieldwork logistics) with harmonization across countries, providing critical insights and practical groundwork to inform the design and implementation of the main study. Building on these foundations, GUIDE has developed a comprehensive set of preparatory processes to ensure cross-national comparability prior to the start of data collection, including harmonized measurement instruments, coordinated sampling framework, and standardized fieldwork strategy, described below.

Harmonized Measurement Instruments

The GUIDE survey will include (core) questionnaires, as well as the possibility of cognitive assessments and the collection of biological data. The GUIDE team selected a core set of well-established, validated, and cross-culturally reliable scales that capture universally relevant aspects of child wellbeing. To promote cultural relevance and child-centeredness, youth advisory boards from multiple countries reviewed the constructs and specific items (see Chap. 5 in this book). This participatory approach strengthens the content validity of the instrument with diverse young respondents. The final questionnaire will be translated using the Translation, Review, Adjudication, Pretesting, Documentation (TRAPD) approach (Harkness et al., 2010), a widely recognized method in cross-national survey research that supports both linguistic and cultural equivalence. Although the focus is on standardization, the design also allows for limited national adaptations when culturally necessary. Furthermore, GUIDE addresses potential question order and framing effects by standardizing the structure and wording of the questionnaire across countries. Ideally, piloting in each national context (including techniques such as randomized question orders) is used to identify and mitigate biases arising from item sequencing or framing. These procedures contribute to measurement equivalence and reduce the risk of context-specific distortions in responses.

As a means of providing valid and equitable comparisons of child development across diverse cultures, GUIDE is considering including non-verbal cognitive assessments to measure fundamental cognitive processes that are less influenced by cultural, linguistic, or educational backgrounds (see Chap. 6 in this book). Similarly, the collection of biological data has been considered, including anthropometric measures (e.g., height and weight), measures of activity level (e.g., with wearables), and biospecimens (e.g., salvia, primary teeth, hair; see Chap. 7 in this book). The collection, storage, and interpretation of biological data require standardized protocols, calibrated instruments, and consistent ethical procedures across countries (see Chaps. 2 and 8 in this book).

Harmonized Sampling Framework

The sampling framework governs the harmonized selection, recruitment, and maintenance of the GUIDE sample. To this end, GUIDE emphasizes the use of strict probability sampling, comparable sampling frames (e.g., national population or birth registers where available), and cohort-specific target sample sizes that are proportional to each country's population. It includes a clearly defined target population and uniform inclusion and exclusion criteria across countries, ensuring that each national sample represents the same conceptual population. Furthermore, GUIDE applies consistent time intervals between survey waves and provides standardized guidelines for handling response and attrition rates, contributing to the methodological consistency needed for valid cross-national comparisons (see Chap. 4 in this book).

Harmonized Fieldwork Strategy

GUIDE aims to standardize key aspects of the fieldwork process, including interviewer training, consent procedures, respondent contact protocols, and the timing of data collection, which are essential to prevent methodological bias across countries. Interviewers are trained using centrally developed materials to ensure consistent understanding and implementation of procedures across countries (see Chap. 3 in this book). A central part of this harmonization effort is the selection of comparable survey modes. GUIDE carefully evaluates the feasibility of different approaches such as face-to-face interviews (CAPI), online self-administered interviews (CAWI), telephone interviews (CATI), or video interviews (CAVI). Ideally, the same mode will be used across all countries to minimize mode-related measurement differences.

The GUIDE Pilot Study

To empirically validate the planned harmonization measures across survey instruments and fieldwork procedures, GUIDE conducted a multi-step pilot study in 2023 in five European countries (Croatia, Finland, France, Ireland, and Slovenia). The pilot aimed to test the feasibility and methodological quality of the survey design under real-life conditions and inform necessary adjustments ahead of Wave 1. Building on this, countries (e.g., Denmark, France, Germany, Italy, Norway, UK) are conducting pilot studies to test the translated instruments and further improve the questionnaires. In all countries, a full-scale dress rehearsal is planned prior to the launch of Wave 1 to simulate the entire data collection process, including probability sampling and recruitment processes, and test the instruments under field conditions (see Chap. 5 in this book).

Regarding the *survey instruments*, a pre-pilot phase used cognitive interviewing techniques with 8-year-old children, their caregivers, and caregivers of young children from diverse cultural backgrounds, to assess whether items were interpreted consistently across national and cultural contexts. An instrument study followed to evaluate the structure, clarity, and psychometric properties of the questionnaires. Results showed that most scales demonstrated high reliability, expected one-factor structures, and satisfactory factor loadings. The questionnaires require further translation and cultural adaptation across all participating countries to ensure consistent interpretation and maintain cross-national comparability.

Concerning *sampling strategies*, the pilot study included an evaluation of recruitment procedures and the composition of the achieved sample. The findings indicated that financial incentives could enhance participant motivation and satisfaction, and that Computer-Assisted Video Interviewing (CAVI) may improve response rates among hard-to-reach groups. These insights point to the importance of harmonizing key recruitment elements, such as incentive structures and survey modes, to reduce the risk of selection bias and support sample comparability across countries.

In terms of *fieldwork implementation*, the pilot assessed the operational feasibility and quality of central fieldwork processes. This included testing interview protocols, translation and adaptation of consent forms and guidelines, deployment of data collection software, and real-time field monitoring. The goal was to identify procedural challenges early on and optimize the fieldwork design to ensure that national implementations follow comparable standards. These insights have been instrumental in refining the fieldwork plan for Wave 1 and supporting GUIDE's aim of achieving consistency across diverse survey contexts (see Chap. 3 in this book).

Maximizing Comparability After Data Collection

Even when questionnaires are harmonized and carefully adapted, cultural or linguistic differences can lead to variations in how respondents interpret and respond to items. Therefore, comparability needs to be tested after data has been collected (van de Vijver et al., 2019). GUIDE plans to apply a range of statistical adjustment methods for post-data collection. The following section focuses primarily on one of these adjustment methods, assessing measurement invariance. Conceptually, measurement invariance implies that a construct carries the same meaning across different groups or time points (e.g., countries, survey waves) indicating the absence of construct and item bias (Jude & Kuger, 2018), which is a fundamental requirement for valid cross-national comparisons in longitudinal studies. Without testing for measurement invariance, observed differences among countries may reflect methodological artifacts rather than true differences in the construct.

Assessing measurement invariance usually involves testing whether key parameters of the measurement model (e.g., factor loadings, item intercepts, residual variances) are equivalent across groups (Meredith, 1993). This examines whether a given scale operates equivalently across groups by testing several levels of invariance (van de Vijver & Leung, 1997; van de Vijver et al., 2019):

- *Configural invariance*: tests whether the same latent construct exists across all countries and whether the same set of items can be used to measure it. If configural invariance is not achieved, it cannot be assumed that respondents in different countries interpret the construct similarly.
- *Metric invariance*: assesses whether the relationship between each item and the underlying construct (i.e., the factor loadings) is equal across countries. In other words, it examines whether each item contributes to the construct to the same extent in all groups. If metric invariance is not achieved, comparisons of relationships among constructs (e.g., regressions or correlations) across countries are

not valid, because the items are not measuring the same underlying construct in different contexts.

- *Scalar invariance*: tests whether the item intercepts are equal, which is a necessary condition for meaningful mean comparisons among countries. Intercepts reflect the baseline level at which respondents begin to endorse an item, assuming they have the same level of the underlying trait. If intercepts differ across countries, it means that some groups tend to systematically agree or disagree more with an item—even if their actual level of the construct is the same. Without scalar invariance, mean differences may therefore reflect systematic response biases (such as cultural tendencies to agree or disagree) rather than true differences on the construct. Achieving full scalar invariance is often challenging in large-scale cross-national studies, but partial invariance approaches may still allow for robust comparisons (Robitzsch & Lüdtke, 2023).

In the context of GUIDE, testing for measurement invariance is a key step to ensure that scales used to assess child wellbeing are psychometrically equivalent across diverse national settings. The standard way to test for measurement invariance is using multi-group confirmatory factor analysis (MG-CFA). MG-CFA is a widely applied method in cross-cultural and longitudinal research (e.g., Wurster, 2022). It involves estimating a sequence of increasingly constrained models to assess whether the measurement structure (e.g., factor loadings and item intercepts) is equivalent across groups, while monitoring changes in model fit to detect potential non-invariance.

It is worth noting that recent literature has raised critical points regarding its limitations, including challenges related to model fit, required sample sizes, and the interpretation of partial invariance (for a recent overview, see Sterner, 2025). For example, this debate surrounds the conventional use of fixed cut-off values in evaluating measurement invariance. Commonly used thresholds such as a change in CFI of less than 0.01 or RMSEA of less than 0.01 have been widely adopted for judging measurement invariance (Putnick & Bornstein, 2016), recent research has highlighted their limitations. Their sensitivity varies depending on factors such as model complexity, sample size, and the presence of cross-loadings (Goretzko et al., 2023). Simulation-based approaches offer an alternative by generating fit index cut-offs that are specific to the model and data conditions under investigation (McNeish, 2023). These methods, while still evolving, hold promises for more precise and context-sensitive invariance testing and may be especially relevant for complex, multi-group studies like GUIDE. For the time being, we recommend that GUIDE continue to rely on the widely used MG-CFA framework, while actively monitoring these methodological developments and assessing their potential integration into future waves of the study.

How to Test for Measurement Invariance: A Case Study Using TIMSS 2019

To illustrate the application of measurement invariance testing, the following case study applies multi-group confirmatory factor analysis (MG-CFA) to assess whether the measurement models of interest function equivalently across countries. MG-CFA provides a structured approach for testing whether participants from different national samples interpret and respond to scale items in statistically comparable ways. Estimating and comparing a sequence of increasingly restrictive models (configural, metric, and scalar invariance) helps determine whether meaningful comparisons of latent constructs can be made across groups. Configural invariance is evaluated based on overall model fit, typically reported with the chi-square statistic (χ^2) and two to four alternative fit indices, such as Root Mean Square Error of Approximation (RMSEA), Standardized Root Mean-square Residual (SRMR), Comparative Fit Index (CFI), and Tucker–Lewis Index (TLI). Metric and scalar invariance are tested by comparing nested models that differ only in specific equality constraints. Changes in fit indices indicate whether the added constraints significantly affect model fit (Putnick & Bornstein, 2016).

The case study uses data from the Trends in International Mathematics and Science Study (TIMSS 2019; Mullis et al., 2020). TIMSS is an international large-scale assessment conducted every four years by the International Association for the Evaluation of Educational Achievement (IEA). The 2019 cycle included fourth- and eighth-grade students from 64 countries and assessed their competencies in mathematics and science, as well as background information on students' learning environments and psychosocial experiences through student questionnaires, making it a valuable secondary resource for testing constructs related to child wellbeing.

TIMSS 2019 initiated offering digital administration to participating countries, reflecting TIMSS's commitment to the future of e-administered large-scale assessments. Consequently, this case study focuses specifically on the subset of data collected through the digital platform, enabling a more relevant and contemporary examination of measurement invariance within a digitally administered context,[2] which aligns well with GUIDE's focus on digitalization in children's lives. To come close to the GUIDE sample (8-year-olds in Wave 1), only the data of fourth graders in TIMSS are analyzed.

TIMSS Case Study Measures

The two constructs selected for this case study, *Sense of Belonging* and *Bullying*, have been examined in previous studies using 2019 TIMSS data. For example,

[2] This subsample of the TIMSS 2019 data, namely the eT19PSI_G4 dataset, only includes responses from students who participated in the Problem Solving and Inquiry (PSI) tasks administered via the digital eTIMSS platform. Consequently, the findings from this analysis are based on a more narrowly defined sample and may not be fully generalizable to the broader population of fourth-grade students assessed in TIMSS 2019 (Fishbein et al., 2018).

Atilgan and Deniz (2023) find scalar invariance for *Sense of Belonging* for 8th-grade students in Turkey, and Sideridis and Alghamdi (2023) find evidence for a multidimensional structure and measurement invariance of *Bullying* across gender for 8th-grade students in Saudi Arabia. Huang et al. (2023) use a framework of item response theory to conclude that the *Sense of Belonging* scale varied considerably across China (Hong Kong), Singapore, Australia, and the USA for grade 4 and grade 8. Focusing on different constructs, others investigate measurement invariance across countries by conducting MG-CFA (Wurster, 2022; Yalçınkaya et al., 2024) or an item response theory (IRT) modeling approach (e.g., Reynolds et al., 2022). By conducting MG-CFA, He et al. (2018) find evidence for metric invariance for *Sense of Belonging*, but with 2015 TIMSS data for 8th-grade students. To our knowledge, no existing study has tested measurement invariance for the constructs *Sense of Belonging* and *Bullying* based on TIMSS 2019 data among fourth-grade students in France, Germany, and Norway—three countries that are preparing to participate in the GUIDE study. TIMSS 2019 assesses "Sense of School Belonging" using five items with a 4-point Likert-type scale ("agree a lot," "agree a little," "disagree a little," "disagree a lot"). The 11-item battery on "Student Bullying" uses a 4-point frequency scale ("never," "a few times a year," "once or twice a month," "at least once a week").

TIMSS Case Study Analyses and Results

Data from France (FRA), Germany (GER), and Norway (NOR) were included in sequential MG-CFA analyses conducted in R (lavaan package; Rosseel, 2012).[3] To prepare for confirmatory modeling, exploratory factor analyses (EFA) were first conducted separately by country. Prior to this, each national dataset was cleansed of missing values via listwise deletion, ensuring complete-case subsamples for the exploration. This step avoided biases due to country-level differences in item nonresponse or imputation strategies. EFAs (principal factor analysis with promax rotation) yielded a unidimensional factor structure for Sense of School Belonging and a two-factor structure for Student Bullying (items 1–7: offline bullying; items 8–10: online bullying), with item 11 being excluded due to substantial but inconsistent cross-loadings across countries (TIMSS & PIRLS International Study Center, 2020). For the confirmatory factor analyses (CFA), the entire available dataset from all three countries was used. Missing values were addressed using Full Information Maximum Likelihood (FIML), which assumes that data are missing at random (MAR) and is

[3] These three countries were selected for both pragmatic and conceptual reasons. First, they are part of the five focus countries emphasized by the editorial team of this volume, and corresponding data were available in the current dataset. Second, they represent a meaningful contrast in terms of child and family policy frameworks as well as levels of reported child wellbeing. For example, Norway is known for its strong welfare state and consistently high scores on child wellbeing indicators, whereas France and Germany follow different policy models and show more mixed outcomes in cross-national comparisons. At the same time, all three are high-income countries in Western Europe, which allows for comparison within a relatively similar socioeconomic context.

robust to item-level nonresponse. This resulted in effective sample sizes of 4,443 (FRA), 3,230 (GER), and 4,188 (NOR) for the Sense of School Belonging scale, and 4,301 (FRA), 3,071 (GER), and 3,985 (NOR) for the Student Bullying scale. The combination of exploratory and confirmatory approaches supports both theory-driven modeling and empirical validation of construct structure—an essential strategy in cross-national research.

For both scales, the results of the invariance analyses support data interpretation at the level of metric invariance, but not at the level of scalar invariance (see Table 9.2). For *Sense of School Belonging*, the unidimensional CFA at the configural level shows a good overall fit of the data to the theoretical measurement model, though the RMSEA slightly exceeds the cut-off for a very good fit as suggested by Hu and Bentler (1999). Model fit decreases somewhat under the assumption of metric invariance yet remains within the acceptable-to-good range across indices. The BIC increases slightly (by 100.18, or less than 0.1%), indicating only a marginal decline in model parsimony and not enough to undermine the results. In contrast, the model assuming scalar invariance shows a substantial deterioration in fit across all indices, suggesting that full scalar invariance cannot be assumed for this scale.

Overall, the fit indices for the two-dimensional CFA at the configural level for *Student Bullying* indicate an acceptable to good model fit, with CFI and TLI on the lower end of the acceptable range, whereas RMSEA and SRMR fall within the good to very good range. Model fit decreases slightly under the assumption of metric invariance, yet RMSEA and SRMR remain well within acceptable thresholds, and the fit can still be considered adequate given the complexity of the two-factor structure. The BIC increases by only 90.58 points, or less than 0.05%, indicating a very small reduction in model fit. Under scalar invariance, the fit further declines, particularly in CFI and RMSEA, whereas SRMR remains acceptable. This suggests that full scalar invariance is questionable, although the fit indices do not drop below minimal acceptability thresholds. Hence, the results do not support strong evidence for scalar invariance in this model.

TIMSS Case Study Discussion

In clear terms, these results support the conclusion that in the three countries under study, the two theoretical dimensions "Sense of School Belonging" and "Student Bullying" can be assessed reliably with the items proposed in the TIMSS 2019 questionnaire. All items contribute to the latent constructs in all countries (same factor structure, i.e., configural invariance) and the items even contribute equally (equal factor loadings in the three countries, i.e., metric invariance). The relations between each item and its latent factor are statistically equivalent in each country. Yet, 8-year-old students in the three countries under study seem to use the answering scale differently (non-invariance of item intercepts, i.e., scalar non-invariance), making it illegitimate to compare items' raw scale scores across countries. Even though scalar invariance seems to be the ultimate goal of cross-national comparison studies, scalar non-invariance is more common than not (Meitinger et al., 2020). A potential

Table 9.2 Fit Indices—Model Evaluation (MG-CFA)

Model	CFI	TLI	RMSEA	SRMR	BIC
Cut-off criteria (Hu & Bentler, 1999)	≥0.95	≥0.95	≤0.06	≤0.08	–
Sense of School Belonging					
Configural invariance	0.972	0.944	0.077	0.023	126,415.405
Metric invariance	0.959	0.947	0.076	0.040	126,515.583
Scalar invariance	0.801	0.807	0.144	0.094	128,468.872
Student Bullying					
Configural invariance	0.942	0.924	0.068	0.038	198,126.186
Metric invariance	0.935	0.926	0.067	0.047	198,216.761
Scalar invariance	0.917	0.917	0.071	0.052	198,640.182

reason is that response styles can vary substantially across countries; for example, students in some countries are more inclined to use the extreme ends of the scales, whereas students in other countries tend to answer more centrally. Translation issues could cause similar problems. Frequency scales (e.g., *never, rarely, sometimes, often, always*) tend to be particularly vulnerable to non-identical translation.

As scalar non-invariance is quite common in cross-national research, several approaches have been developed to address it. One such approach involves conducting latent mean comparisons under the assumption of partial invariance of the latent construct. This means that although some parameters (typically item intercepts, i.e., mean estimates, or residual variances) are allowed to vary across countries, others are constrained to be equal. The idea is to acknowledge that not all items function equivalently across groups, and instead of discarding the entire scale, focus the analysis on those items that do show invariance. Implementing this strategy requires a thorough investigation of potential sources of partial non-invariance for each analysis and the use of latent variable models that explicitly account for these differences. Although the results from these models can be informative, they should be interpreted with caution and interpretation should rely more heavily on aspects that are captured in invariant items (and less on variant items) of the latent construct.

In large-scale studies, central data agencies often perform these advanced analyses for questionnaire constructs and provide scaled scores—based either on Item Response Theory (IRT) or Classical Test Theory (CTT)—alongside the released data. For example, TIMSS 2019 constructed such scales using IRT methods, specifically the Rasch partial credit model (Masters & Wright, 1997). TIMSS 2015 illustrates this scaling approach with the "Sense of Belonging" scale for eighth graders (Martin et al., 2017).

If scalar invariance cannot be fully established, researchers may alternatively adjust their analytic focus. Instead of directly comparing mean levels of constructs such as student bullying across countries, they can examine within-country group differences or associations between variables. For instance, gender differences in reported sense of school belonging could be analyzed separately within each country, or correlations between students' socioeconomic status and bullying could be explored on a country-by-country basis. This strategy enables the identification of meaningful, country-specific patterns even when direct cross-country mean comparisons are not justified. However, such findings should not be interpreted as absolute differences between countries, but rather as context-specific insights valid within each national sample.

Conclusion: Contribution to Evidence-Based Policies

Ensuring cross-nationally comparable data is one of the greatest challenges in cross-national survey research. In the GUIDE study, which aims to capture child wellbeing across Europe, this challenge extends beyond aligning timelines or translating questionnaires. Cultural, linguistic, and contextual differences can affect how concepts are understood, how questions are answered, and how responses are interpreted. If such biases remain undetected, they may distort the findings and result in misleading conclusions. GUIDE therefore applies a range of procedures to promote comparability, including harmonized instrument development, cognitive testing, and statistical analyses of measurement invariance. These efforts help to ensure that observed differences among countries reflect true variation in children's lives rather than artifacts of measurement.

Testing for measurement invariance is a crucial step in this process. Without it, cross-national comparisons risk being invalid. When different groups interpret or respond to items differently, *group means* cannot be meaningfully compared. Statistical models such as multiple-group confirmatory factor analysis allow for a structured assessment of whether the same constructs are measured in the same way. If scalar invariance is established, researchers can compare latent means with confidence. At the same time, it should be acknowledged that the practice of evaluating measurement invariance based on fixed cut-off criteria is subject to growing critique. Recent methodological work has highlighted that such thresholds may not generalize across different models, sample sizes, or item characteristics, prompting calls for more flexible, simulation-based approaches. Although a new standard has yet to be established, it is important that studies like GUIDE remain attentive to these developments and assess their potential for future application. The importance of comparability in GUIDE lies in its broader objective. The study is designed to generate robust evidence to guide policy decisions that improve the wellbeing of children and adolescents across Europe. Without valid comparisons, it is impossible to identify patterns, detect inequalities, or design interventions that respond to actual needs. In this sense, methodological precision is not a technical detail but a prerequisite for effective, evidence-based policymaking.

This chapter outlines the major challenges and methodological strategies involved in achieving comparability in large-scale cross-national studies. It highlights why measurement invariance is essential, how it can be tested, and what the implications are when it is not ensured. By illustrating these issues in the context of child wellbeing, the chapter aims to serve as a resource for researchers working with GUIDE or similar datasets. At the same time, it acknowledges that the field is evolving. New tools and critiques are emerging that question the assumptions of earlier methods. GUIDE, as an ambitious and long-term cross-national effort, should remain responsive to these developments to ensure that the findings continue to meet the highest standards of validity and usefulness.

References

Atılgan, M., & Deniz, K. Z. (2023). Investigation of the measurement invariance of affective characteristics related to TIMSS 2019 mathematics achievement by gender. *Eğitimde ve Psikolojide Ölçme ve Değerlendirme Dergisi = Journal of Measurement and Evaluation in Education and Psychology, 14*(3), 185–199. https://doi.org/10.21031/epod.1221365

Benítez, I., van de Vijver, F., & Padilla, J. L. (2022). A mixed methods approach to the analysis of bias in cross-cultural studies. *Sociological Methods & Research, 51*(1), 237–270. https://doi.org/10.1177/0049124119852390

Boeije, H., & Willis, G. (2013). The Cognitive Interviewing Reporting Framework (CIRF): Towards the harmonization of cognitive testing reports. *Methodology: European Journal of Research Methods for the Behavioral and Social Sciences, 9*(3), 87–95. https://doi.org/10.1027/1614-2241/a000075

Davidov, E., Meuleman, B., Cieciuch, J., Schmidt, P., & Billiet, J. (2014). Measurement equivalence in cross-national research. *Annual Review of Sociology, 40*(1), 55–75. https://doi.org/10.1146/annurev-soc-071913-043137

Desa, D., van de Vijver, F., Carstens, R., & Schulz, W. (2018). Measurement invariance in international large-scale assessments: Integrating theory and method. In T. P. Johnson, B.-E. Pennell, I. A. L. Stoop, & B. Dorer (Eds.), *Advances in comparative survey methodology* (pp. 881–910). Wiley.

Eremenco, S. L., Cella, D., & Arnold, B. J. (2005). A comprehensive method for the translation and cross-cultural validation of health status questionnaires. *Evaluation & the Health Professions, 28*(2), 212–232. https://doi.org/10.1177/0163278705275342

Exenberger, S., Banzer, R., Christy, J., Höfer, S., & Juen, B. (2019). Eastern and Western children's voices on their well-being. *Child Indicators Research, 12*, 747–768. https://doi.org/10.1007/s12187-018-9541-8

Fishbein, B., Martin, M. O., Mullis, I. V. S., & Foy, P. (2018). The TIMSS 2019 item equivalence study: Examining mode effects for computer-based assessment and implications for measuring trends. *Large-Scale Assessments in Education, 6*(1), Article 11. https://doi.org/10.1186/s40536-018-0064-z

Fitzgerald, R., Widdop, S., Gray, M., & Collins, D. (2009, March). *Testing for equivalence using cross-national cognitive interviewing* (Working Paper Series No. 01). Centre for Comparative Social Surveys, City University London.

Goretzko, D., Siemund, K., & Sterner, P. (2023). Evaluating model fit of measurement models in confirmatory factor analysis. *Educational and Psychological Measurement, 84*(1), 123–144.

Harkness, J. A., Villar, A., & Edwards, B. (2010). Translation, adaptation, and design. In J. A. Harkness, M. Braun, B. Edwards, T. P. Johnson, L. E. Lyberg, P. P. Mohler, B.-E. Pennell, & T. W. Smith (Eds.), *Survey methods in multinational, multiregional, and multicultural contexts* (pp. 115–140). Wiley.

Harzing, A.-W. (2006). Response styles in cross-national survey research: A 26-country study. *International Journal of Cross Cultural Management, 6*(2), 243–266. https://doi.org/10.1177/1470595806066332

He, J., Barrera-Pedemonte, F., & Buchholz, J. (2018). Cross-cultural comparability of noncognitive constructs in TIMSS and PISA. *Assessment in Education: Principles, Policy & Practice, 26*(4), 369–385.

He, J., & van de Vijver, F. J. R. (2012). Bias and equivalence in cross-cultural research. *Online Readings in Psychology and Culture, 2*(2), Article 8. https://doi.org/10.9707/2307-0919.1111

Huang, J., Dong, Y., Han, C., & Wang, X. (2023). Evaluating the language- and culture-related construct-irrelevant variance and reliability of the Sense of School Belonging Scale: Suggestions for revision. *Journal of Psychoeducational Assessment, 41*(8), 852–871. https://doi.org/10.1177/07342829231189319

Hu, L.-T., & Bentler, P. M. (1999). Cutoff criteria for fit indexes in covariance structure analysis: Conventional criteria versus new alternatives. *Structural Equation Modeling, 6*(1), 1–55. https://doi.org/10.1080/10705519909540118

Johnson, T. P., & van de Vijver, F. J. R. (2003). Social desirability in cross-cultural research. In J. A. Harkness, F. J. R. van de Vijver, & PPh. Mohler (Eds.), *Cross-cultural survey methods* (pp. 195–204). Wiley.

Jude, N., & Kuger, S. (2018). *Questionnaire development and design for international large-scale assessments (ILSAs): Current practice, challenges, and recommendations*. National Academy of

Education. http://naeducation.org/wp-content/uploads/2018/04/Jude-and-Kuger-2018-FINAL.pdf

Kitayama, S., Duffy, S., & Uchida, Y. (2007). Self as cultural mode of being. In S. Kitayama & D. Cohen (Eds.), *Handbook of cultural psychology* (pp. 136–173). Guilford Press.

Kitayama, S., & Markus, H. R. (2000). The pursuit of happiness and the realization of sympathy: Cultural patterns of self, social relations, and well-being. In E. Diener & E. M. Suh (Eds.), *Culture and subjective well-being* (pp. 113–161). MIT Press.

Kitayama, S., Markus, H. R., & Kurokawa, M. (2000). Culture, emotion, and well-being: Good feelings in Japan and the United States. *Cognition & Emotion, 14*(1), 93–124. https://doi.org/10.1080/026999300379003

Konca, A. S. (2022). Digital technology usage of young children: Screen time and families. *Early Childhood Education Journal, 50*(7), 1097–1108. https://doi.org/10.1007/s10643-021-01245-7

Korsnakova, P., & Dept, S. (2020). Translation: The preparation of national language versions of assessment instruments. In T. Nilsen, A. Stancel-Piątak, J.-E. Gustafsson, & B. Yang Hansen (Eds.), *Reliability and validity of international large-scale assessment: Understanding IEA's comparative studies of student achievement* (pp. 85–111). Springer. https://doi.org/10.1007/978-3-030-53081-5_6

Krähenbühl, S., & Blades, M. (2006). The effect of question repetition within interviews on young children's eyewitness recall. *Journal of Experimental Child Psychology, 94*(1), 57–67. https://doi.org/10.1016/j.jecp.2005.12.002

Martin, M. O., Mullis, I. V. S., Hooper, M., Yin, L., Foy, P., & Palazzo, L. (2017). Creating and interpreting the TIMSS 2015 context questionnaire scales. In M. O. Martin, I. V. S. Mullis, & M. Hooper (Eds.), *Methods and procedures in TIMSS 2015* (Chap. 15). TIMSS & PIRLS International Study Center, Lynch School of Education and Human Development, Boston College.

Masters, G. N., & Wright, B. D. (1997). The partial credit model. In W. J. van der Linden & R. K. Hambleton (Eds.), *Handbook of modern item response theory* (pp. 101–121). Springer.

McNeish, D. (2023). Dynamic fit index cutoffs for categorical factor analysis with Likert-type, ordinal, or binary responses. *American Psychologist, 78*(9), 1061–1075. https://doi.org/10.1037/amp0001213

Meitinger, K., Davidov, E., Schmidt, P., & Braun, M. (2020). Measurement invariance: Testing for it and explaining why it is absent. *Survey Research Methods, 14*(4), 345–349. https://doi.org/10.18148/srm/2020.v14i4.7655

Meredith, W. (1993). Measurement invariance, factor analysis and factorial invariance. *Psychometrika, 58*(4), 525–543. https://doi.org/10.1007/BF02294825

Mullis, I. V. S., Martin, M. O., Foy, P., Kelly, D. L., & Fishbein, B. (2020). *TIMSS 2019 international results in mathematics and science*. TIMSS & PIRLS International Study Center, Lynch School of Education and Human Development, Boston College, & International Association for the Evaluation of Educational Achievement. https://www.iea.nl/sites/default/files/2021-01/TIMSS%202019-International-Results-in-Mathematics-and-Science.pdf

Putnick, D. L., & Bornstein, M. H. (2016). Measurement invariance conventions and reporting: The state of the art and future directions for psychological research. *Developmental Review, 41*, 71–90. https://doi.org/10.1016/j.dr.2016.06.004

Reynolds, K., Khorramdel, L., & von Davier, M. (2022). Can students' attitudes towards mathematics and science be compared across countries? Evidence from measurement invariance modeling in TIMSS 2019. *Studies in Educational Evaluation, 74*, Article 101183. https://doi.org/10.1016/j.stueduc.2022.101183

Rickwood, D. J., & Coleman-Rose, C. L. (2023). The effect of survey administration mode on youth mental health measures: Social desirability bias and sensitive questions. *Heliyon, 9*(9), Article e19364. https://doi.org/10.1016/j.heliyon.2023.e19364

Robitzsch, A., & Lüdtke, O. (2023). Why full, partial, or approximate measurement invariance are not a prerequisite for meaningful and valid group comparisons. *Structural Equation Modeling: A Multidisciplinary Journal, 30*(6), 859–870. https://doi.org/10.1080/10705511.2023.2197303

Rosseel, Y. (2012). lavaan: An R package for structural equation modeling. *Journal of Statistical Software, 48*(2), 1–36. https://doi.org/10.18637/jss.v048.i02

Rutkowski, L., & Svetina, D. (2014). Assessing the hypothesis of measurement invariance in the context of large-scale international surveys. *Educational and Psychological Measurement, 74*(1), 31–57.

Sideridis, G., & Alghamdi, M. H. (2023). Bullying in middle school: Evidence for a multidimensional structure and measurement invariance across gender. *Children, 10*(5), Article 873. https://doi.org/10.3390/children10050873

Smith, P. B., & Fischer, R. (2008). Acquiescence, extreme response bias and culture: A multilevel analysis. In F. J. R. van de Vijver, D. A. van Hemert, & Y. H. Poortinga (Eds.), *Multilevel analysis of individuals and cultures* (pp. 285–314). Taylor & Francis Group/Lawrence Erlbaum Associates.

Sterner, P. (2025). *On the investigation of measurement invariance: New developments and a causal framework for future research* (Doctoral dissertation, Ludwig-Maximilians-Universität München). LMU München. https://doi.org/10.5282/edoc.34864

TIMSS & PIRLS International Study Center. (2020). *IEA's Trends in International Mathematics and Science Study (TIMSS) 2019: Grade 4 student questionnaire*. International Association for the Evaluation of Educational Achievement & Lynch School of Education and Human Development, Boston College. https://timssandpirls.bc.edu/timss2019/questionnaires/pdf/T19_StuQ_4.pdf

Uchida, Y., Norasakkunkit, V., & Kitayama, S. (2004). Cultural constructions of happiness: Theory and empirical evidence. *Journal of Happiness Studies, 5*(3), 223–239. https://doi.org/10.1007/s10902-004-8785-9

van de Vijver, F. J. R. (2018). Towards an integrated framework of bias in noncognitive assessment in international large-scale studies: Challenges and prospects. *Educational Measurement: Issues and Practice, 37*(4), 49–56. https://doi.org/10.1111/emip.12227

van de Vijver, F. J. R., Jude, N., & Kuger, S. (2019). Challenges in international large-scale educational surveys. In *The SAGE handbook of comparative studies in education* (pp. 83–102). SAGE Publications.

van de Vijver, F. J. R., & Leung, K. (1997). Methods and data analysis of comparative research. In *Handbook of cross-cultural psychology* (Vol. 1, pp. 257–300). Allyn & Bacon.

van de Vijver, F. J. R., & Poortinga, Y. H. (1997). Towards an integrated analysis of bias in cross-cultural assessment. *European Journal of Psychological Assessment, 13*(1), 29–37.

Willis, G. B. (2005). *Cognitive interviewing: A tool for improving questionnaire design*. Sage.

Wurster, S. (2022). Measurement invariance of non-cognitive measures in TIMSS across countries and across time: An application and comparison of multigroup confirmatory factor analysis, Bayesian approximate measurement invariance, and alignment optimization approach. *Studies in Educational Evaluation, 73*, Article 101143. https://doi.org/10.1016/j.stueduc.2022.101143

Yalçınkaya, M., Atılgan, H., Daşcıoğlu, S., & Aydın, B. (2024). The eTIMSS and TIMSS measurement invariance study: Multigroup factor analyses and differential item functioning analyses with the 2019 cycle. *Eğitimde ve Psikolojide Ölçme ve Değerlendirme Dergisi = Journal of Measurement and Evaluation in Education and Psychology, 15*(2), 94–119. https://doi.org/10.21031/epod.1426739

Zavala-Rojas, D., Sorato, D., Hareide, L., & Hofland, K. (2022). The multilingual corpus of survey questionnaires: A tool for refining survey translation. *Meta: Journal des traducteurs, 67*(1), 71–93. https://doi.org/10.7202/1092191ar

Sabine Düval (Ph.D.) is a senior researcher at the German Youth Institute (DJI) and guest researcher at the Federal Institute for Population Research (BiB). She specializes in family sociology and quantitative methods of empirical social research, contributing to international comparability, sampling, and recruitment strategies in the Horizon Europe project Growing Up in Digital Europe Preparation Phase (GUIDEPREP).

Susanne Kuger (Ph.D.) is a professor of Empirical Social and Educational Research in Childhood and Adolescence at LMU Munich, Germany, and Research Director at the German Youth Institute (DJI). She specializes in large-scale assessments, focusing on educational environments and learning outcomes, advancing quantitative methods, and innovative designs in international comparative studies.

Lynda M. Sagrestano (Ph.D.) is a senior researcher at the German Youth Institute (DJI). She specializes in studying the impact of contextual and psychosocial factors on mental health and wellbeing, especially among marginalized youth and families.

Chapter 10
Making Ends Meet: Funding and National Frameworks of Cross-National Cohort Studies

Giovanni Righetto, Giulio Ecchia, and Enrico Elefante

Introduction

Growing Up in Digital Europe (GUIDE) is a novel longitudinal study aimed at generating high-quality, harmonized data on child and youth development across European countries. It represents the first Europe-wide cohort infrastructure focused on understanding how digitalization, social change, and economic inequality shape children's well-being and life trajectories. By following children over time, GUIDE provides researchers and policymakers with a unique evidence base to design and evaluate policies that promote inclusive, sustainable development. This chapter examines the financial foundations and funding strategies required to ensure the long-term sustainability of a large-scale infrastructure. In doing so, it highlights both the strategic importance of investing in child-focused research and the lessons that can be drawn from comparable initiatives such as SHARE and ESS.

GUIDE's Socioeconomic Landscape

This section examines the socioeconomic factors influencing GUIDE, emphasizing the importance of investing in children's well-being, aligning with global frameworks such as the Sustainable Development Goals (SDGs), and analyzing how GUIDE can influence public policy, health, and economic growth.

G. Righetto (✉) · G. Ecchia
Department of Economics, University of Bologna, Bologna, Italy
e-mail: giovannirighetto7@gmail.com

E. Elefante
Italian Youth Agency, Rome, Italy

L. K. Taylor et al. (eds.), *Growing Up in Digital Europe*, Springer Series on Child and Family Studies, https://doi.org/10.1007/978-3-032-30592-3_10

The socioeconomic environment in which GUIDE operates is characterized by significant disparities in income, education, and access to resources. In several regions across Europe, socioeconomic inequalities persist, particularly affecting marginalized communities and vulnerable populations such as rural children and those from lower-income families. According to studies compiled by UNICEF (Richardson et al., 2020) and the OECD (OECD, 2015, 2019), these disparities are associated with long-term negative impacts on children's well-being, limiting their access to quality education, healthcare, and social services. GUIDE aims to address these disparities by developing a comprehensive dataset to capture these socioeconomic dimensions and the impact on child development across different countries.

GUIDE's objectives are aligned with international efforts such as the 2030 Agenda for Sustainable Development, particularly focusing on goals related to reducing inequalities, ensuring inclusive education, and promoting good health and well-being. By positioning itself within these global efforts, GUIDE contributes not only to scientific knowledge but also to the achievement of policy targets aimed at fostering sustainable and equitable development.

GUIDE's Socioeconomic Impact

The socioeconomic impact of GUIDE is anticipated to be significant and multidimensional, delivering benefits across several societal sectors. Following Florio (2019), research conducted by Ecchia et al. (2021) suggests that the advantages of utilizing longitudinal survey infrastructures such as GUIDE can be grouped into four primary areas:

- *Value and Efficiency Gains for Researchers*: GUIDE will streamline research by providing a sophisticated infrastructure for collecting and analyzing data on child well-being (e.g., data on breastfeeding rates, immunization, parent and child nutrition, and mental health indicators). This will enhance research efficiency, reduce redundancy, and encourage cross-national and interdisciplinary collaboration.
- *Knowledge Output*: The longitudinal data generated by GUIDE will significantly expand the understanding of child well-being across Europe. The depth of this data will reveal key trends and correlations that cross-sectional studies cannot detect. For example, studies have shown that children living in poverty are more likely to face barriers to education and health services, creating cycles of disadvantage that last into adulthood. By tracking changes over time, GUIDE will inform policies designed to mitigate these effects.
- *Human Capital Growth*: Human capital refers to the skills, knowledge, and experiences possessed by individuals which are a key factor for economic growth and societal well-being. Children who grow up in socioeconomic disadvantage often face barriers that limit their access to educational opportunities and healthcare, resulting in reduced economic prospects later in life (OECD, 2015, 2019). Investments in early childhood education have been shown to yield high returns

in terms of human capital accumulation, with studies showing that children who receive quality education in their early years are more likely to complete higher levels of education and secure better-paying jobs as adults (Conti & Gupta, 2024). Center-based programs such as Head Start (US) and Sure Start (UK) demonstrate long-term benefits in education, health, and employment, especially for disadvantaged children (Conti & Gupta, 2024). GUIDE will provide policymakers with the data needed to understand these links better, identify barriers and the critical points in a child's development where interventions can have the most significant long-term effects, and design interventions that foster the development of strong human capital from early childhood identity.

- *Benefits to End-Users*: One of the most significant impacts of GUIDE will be on its end-users—policymakers, children, and young people. The data and insights generated by the project will empower policymakers to design more effective interventions aimed at improving child well being, thereby addressing socioeconomic inequalities. For children and young people, the benefits of GUIDE's findings are direct and profound. GUIDE data will lead to better educational outcomes, improved mental and physical health, and enhanced social participation, over time resulting in a more equitable and prosperous society, where every child can reach their full potential.

Methodological Added Value

GUIDE's methodological approach, particularly its longitudinal design, is one of the project's core strengths. This approach allows researchers to track the developmental trajectories of children over time, offering a unique opportunity to study the dynamic nature of child development in different socioeconomic contexts. GUIDE's design allows for the examination of disruptive events, such as the COVID-19 pandemic, wars, or climate phenomena, and their differential impacts on child development. This will enable researchers to isolate the effects of such events from confounding variables, providing clearer insights into how crises impact child well-being and future mitigation efforts.

Long-Term Benefits

By tracking children through to adulthood, GUIDE will shed light on the intergenerational impacts of socioeconomic conditions, highlighting how the experiences of one generation affect the well being of the next. Cost-benefit analyses estimate that the availability of new data provided by GUIDE could lead to improvements in the effectiveness of European spending on child and youth well being. Specifically, an efficiency improvement of around €1 in every €16,000 spent would be sufficient for the benefits of GUIDE to outweigh its costs (Ecchia et al., 2024).

GUIDE's Imperative: Investing in Children

Investing in children's well-being is central to GUIDE's mission and is increasingly recognized as a critical component of broader societal development. Strategic investments in children's education, health, and social inclusion are essential for fostering resilient and productive communities. Children who receive strong support in their early years, particularly in terms of education and healthcare, are more likely to become productive members of society, driving innovation and contributing to sustainable economic development (Cunha et al., 2006). A randomized evaluation of the Irish *Preparing for Life* program demonstrated that providing intensive parenting support from pregnancy to age five improved cognitive outcomes by two-thirds of a standard deviation and socioemotional outcomes by one-quarter. These effects were particularly pronounced for firstborns and children from lower-resource households, effectively narrowing the socioeconomic gap in early skills acquisition (Doyle, 2020).

As of 2025, nearly one in four children in the European Union—approximately 24%—are at risk of poverty or social exclusion (Eurostat, 2024). Across Europe, children from marginalized communities, including those from low-income families, ethnic minorities, and rural populations, face systemic barriers to accessing quality education, healthcare, and social services. Economic disparities are strongly correlated with negative outcomes in childhood, including lower educational attainment, poorer health, and reduced social mobility (Chetty et al., 2014). Children from low-income backgrounds can grow up lacking stimulation and basic investments, which may lead to developmental deficits that are difficult, if not impossible, to reverse later in life without intervention (Attanasio et al., 2022). Children from lower-income households are less likely to complete secondary education, and those who do often face limited opportunities for higher education or stable employment. This disparity reflects the persistent effects of early poverty, which influence adult outcomes—including education, employment, and health—even after controlling for later-life circumstances (Duncan et al., 2010).

Children in lower-income households are significantly more likely to experience poor health outcomes, including chronic illnesses, malnutrition, and delayed development. These are often compounded by inadequate housing, limited access to healthcare, and exposure to environmental hazards. Economic research shows that early-life disadvantages—ranging from maternal stress to pollution—can have permanent effects on children's cognitive and physical development (Almond et al., 2018). GUIDE will help track these long-term consequences, such as asthma, obesity, and reduced school performance, that disproportionately affect disadvantaged children (Aizer & Currie, 2019; Currie & Almond, 2011). Intergenerational transmission of health inequality, such as parental health behaviors, stress, and socioeconomic conditions, strongly influences children's developmental trajectories. Cunha and Heckman (2007) argue that health, like education, is subject to dynamic complementarities—early advantages (or disadvantages) compound over time.

Mental health disorders impose an estimated cost of 2.5% of the GDP in the US and 3.5% of the GDP in Europe (Kiessling & Norris, 2020); also, recent evidence exposed a progressive worsening of general mental conditions during the last decade, especially for young people (Braghieri et al., 2022). Children living in poverty or experiencing social exclusion are at a higher risk of developing mental health issues, such as anxiety, depression, and behavioral disorders (Almond et al., 2018). A large-scale study conducted in France during the COVID-19 pandemic found that children from lower socioeconomic backgrounds were significantly more likely to exhibit mental health problems, including increased symptoms of hyperactivity/inattention and emotional distress. This elevated risk was associated with factors such as prior low family socioeconomic status and a decline in income during the pandemic, highlighting the compounded effects of economic disadvantage on child mental health (Moulin et al., 2023).

Investing in the Digital Divide

One of the critical challenges that GUIDE seeks to address is the growing digital divide, which has become evident across Europe in recent years. Access to and healthy use of technologies have been shown to be fundamental for children's capability to develop cognitive skills (Cristia et al., 2017; Malamud & Pop-Eleches, 2011). Findings from longitudinal studies such as The French Longitudinal Study of Children (ELFE, 2025) and Growing Up in Ireland (GUI; Quail et al., 2011) show that children's digital media exposure is strongly linked to family income and parental education levels, with children from more disadvantaged backgrounds experiencing greater risks of overuse or unsupervised access.

During the COVID-19 pandemic, these inequalities were further exacerbated: in Ireland, for example, over 50% of children from lower-income families reported difficulty engaging with online learning due to lack of devices or internet access (Ecchia et al., 2024). A growing body of economic research emphasizes that access to digital tools enhances the effectiveness of human capital accumulation, particularly when technology complements high-quality instruction and learning environments. Recent work by Agostinelli et al. (2022) found that unequal access to digital technology during the pandemic significantly contributed to the widening of skill gaps among children, especially in early education, where developmental windows are most sensitive. Their structural model suggests that the absence of digital learning tools among disadvantaged groups could have long-lasting effects on earnings and intergenerational mobility. This digital divide disproportionately affects children from lower-income families, who are less likely to have access to the technology needed for remote learning (Bulman & Fairlie, 2016). As a result, these children faced greater educational setbacks during the pandemic compared to their more affluent peers; in turn, these difficulties widened the social class achievement gap (Goudeau et al., 2021).

Investing in Societal Development and Economic Growth

Investing in children's well-being is not only a moral imperative but also an essential driver of societal development and economic growth. GUIDE emphasizes the long-term economic benefits of investing in child development, particularly in terms of human capital formation. By improving access to quality education, healthcare, and social services, societies can cultivate a more skilled, healthy, and productive workforce, which is essential for sustained economic growth.

Numerous studies have demonstrated a strong correlation between early childhood development and economic prosperity. For example, children who receive adequate healthcare and education are more likely to become productive adults who contribute positively to the economy (Felfe & Lalive, 2018). Conversely, childhood poverty has significant long-term economic consequences, not only for the individuals affected but also for society. Children who grow up in poverty are more likely to experience academic difficulties, limiting their ability to secure stable, well-paying jobs later in life. Failing to invest in children's well-being leads to higher social welfare costs, as those who grow up in poverty are more likely to experience unemployment, poor health, and social exclusion later in life (Almond et al., 2018), which places additional strain on social welfare systems (Cunha et al., 2006).

GUIDE data will provide the evidence base needed to advocate for increased public investment in children, demonstrating the long-term returns on such investments for both individuals and society. By addressing the needs of the most vulnerable children, these policies will help reduce socioeconomic inequalities, fostering a more equitable distribution of resources and opportunities.

International Policy Implications and Recommendations

GUIDE is not only shaped by national contexts but also operates within a broader framework of European Union and international policies focused on child well-being, education, and social inclusion. The EU has long recognized the importance of addressing socioeconomic disparities among children, as reflected in policies such as the European Pillar of Social Rights, which emphasizes equal opportunities for all children regardless of socioeconomic background. One key initiative under this Pillar is the Child Guarantee, which aims to ensure that every child in the EU has access to healthcare, education, childcare, housing, and nutrition, particularly those in vulnerable situations. EUROSTAT data shows that nearly 24.2% of children in the EU were at risk of poverty or social exclusion (Eurostat, 2024). GUIDE's longitudinal approach will allow policymakers to track progress toward the Child Guarantee goals over time, offering insights into where additional resources and interventions are needed.

In addition to European policies, GUIDE aligns with the United Nations Sustainable Development Goals (SDGs), particularly Goal 1 (No Poverty), Goal 3 (Good

Health and Well being), and Goal 4 (Quality Education). These global goals emphasize the importance of reducing inequalities, ensuring access to healthcare and education for all children, and promoting inclusive and equitable societies. GUIDE's findings will contribute to global efforts to monitor progress toward these goals, providing data that can inform both national and cross-national strategies for child development.

Furthermore, GUIDE will play a key role in supporting the European Education Area (EEA), which aims to create a space where quality education and training are accessible to all across Europe. By providing data on how socioeconomic factors influence educational outcomes, GUIDE will help shape policies that ensure all children, regardless of their background, can benefit from the opportunities provided by the EEA. This includes addressing barriers such as the digital divide, regional disparities, and socioeconomic inequalities, all of which can hinder children's access to quality education.

Improving child well-being requires an integrated policy approach that addresses multiple dimensions of a child's life, including education, health, family support, and social inclusion. GUIDE's research will provide the evidence base needed to advocate for such an approach, demonstrating the interconnectedness of these factors and the importance of addressing them simultaneously (see Chap. 1 in this book). A comprehensive, whole-of-society and whole-of-government approach is essential—one that harnesses diverse expertise, aligns policies with children's needs and expectations, and ensures coordinated efforts among key stakeholders, including governments, service providers, educators, and families (OECD, 2025).

Box 10.1: Socioeconomic Inequalities in Education and Health: The Case of Italy

In Italy, as in many European countries, childhood poverty is linked to higher rates of unemployment and social exclusion in adulthood. A 2021 study by Caritas Italy (Caritas, 2021) found that children who grow up in poverty are three times more likely to experience poverty as adults, perpetuating a cycle of disadvantage that is difficult to break without targeted interventions.

In Italy, significant regional differences in income, education, and healthcare services exist between the northern and southern parts of the country. ISTAT data reveals that children growing up in southern regions, such as Calabria and Sicily, are more likely to face economic hardship and have limited access to high-quality education and healthcare compared to their peers in wealthier northern regions like Lombardy and Emilia-Romagna (ISTAT, 2024).

One stark example of this is the school dropout rate, which is notably higher in southern Italy. According to a 2022 report from Save the Children Italy, nearly 18% of students in southern regions leave school early, compared to just 11% in the north. This educational disparity is closely linked to the socioeconomic conditions of the families in these areas, where high unemployment rates and low household incomes limit access to educational resources. GUIDE's longitudinal approach will provide the data needed to track how these regional disparities evolve, offering policymakers insights into how targeted educational interventions could reduce dropout rates and improve overall educational outcomes. Another issue highlighted during the COVID-19 pandemic is the importance of digital infrastructure for education, as schools shifted to remote learning. However, not all children were equally equipped to handle this transition. In Italy, ISTAT reported that nearly 12% of households with children did not have access to a computer or reliable internet connection during the pandemic, with the percentage rising to 20% in southern regions (ISTAT, 2024).

In terms of healthcare, children in southern Italy also face greater challenges. The availability of healthcare services in these regions is often more limited, with fewer hospitals and specialized pediatric services. ISTAT data indicates that children in poorer southern regions are more likely to suffer from chronic health conditions, such as obesity and asthma, which are exacerbated by environmental and socioeconomic factors (ISTAT, 2024). Italy, with its extensive but regionally uneven welfare system, provides a unique case study for understanding how public policies can either alleviate or exacerbate the effects of poverty on children. By analyzing these dynamics, GUIDE will help inform the development of more effective national and regional policies that improve access to healthcare, promote economic mobility, and reduce poverty rates in future generations, ensuring that all can flourish.

GUIDE's Financial Strategies: Evidence from SHARE and ESS

This section examines the financial frameworks of two major research infrastructures—Survey of Health, Aging, and Retirement in Europe (SHARE; Börsch-Supan et al., 2019, 2020, 2021, 2022, 2023, 2024) and European Social Survey (ESS; Davidov et al., 2008)—to draw insights relevant to the sustainable financing of GUIDE (see Box 10.2). By analyzing the financial strategies of these successful research infrastructures, GUIDE can develop a robust and sustainable financial plan that ensures its long-term viability and impact.

Box 10.2: Survey of Health, Aging, and Retirement in Europe (SHARE)

SHARE is a research infrastructure that studies the effects of health, social, economic, and environmental policies over the life-course of European citizens and beyond. SHARE became an ERIC in 2011, and 16 countries are ERIC members. It is the largest pan-European social science panel study providing cross-nationally comparable longitudinal data which allows insights into health and socioeconomic living conditions of Europeans, both for scientists and policymakers.

Budget: (2023 example) €7–8 M

DG EMPL support: ~€750 k

Administrative (membership) fees: ~€280 k

Central coordination (from Germany's BMBF): ~€2.0 M

Project grants (EU and US): ~€3.5 M

Funding Sources: SHARE is publicly funded, and sources can be grouped into three categories:

National contributions (member countries): **~50%**

Most of the survey costs are covered by national ministries or research councils. In many cases, member countries transfer these funds to SHARE-ERIC, which manages the procurement of national survey agencies.

European Commission (DG EMPL and DG RTD): **~35%**

The European Commission contributes significantly, Employment, Social Affairs and Inclusion (DG EMPL) funds countries unable to fully finance participation through EUCOV mechanism (e.g., BG, CY, FI, LT, LV, MT, RO, SK, plus EE, ES, GR, PT as "crisis countries"). Additionally, Research and Innovation (DG RTD) supports project grants such as SHARE-COHESION and SHARE COVID-19.

Grants from other sources (e.g., US National Institute on Aging): **~15%**

Project-specific funds come from international research programs. For instance, in 2023, a US NIA grant supported the SHARE-HCAP module on cognitive impairment.

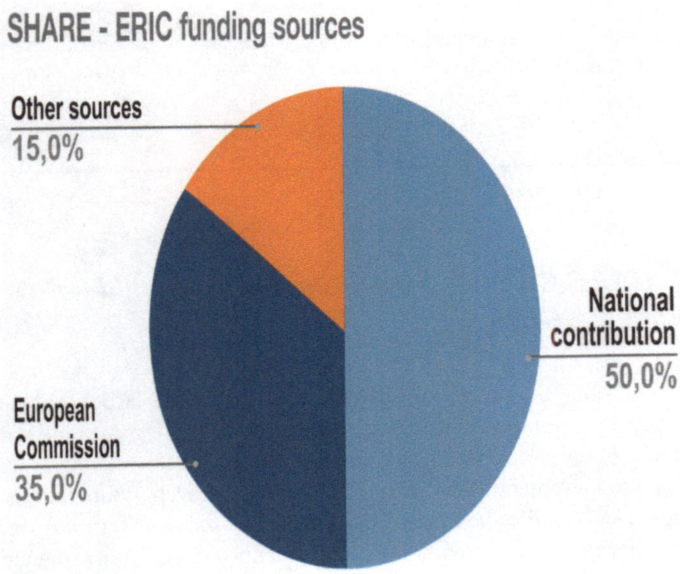

Outputs: As of 2023, SHARE conducted over 600,000 in-depth interviews across 28 European countries and Israel, supported by over €150 million raised through national contributions and European or international grants. SHARE has expanded incrementally across survey waves; participation varies by wave due to funding, infrastructure readiness, and EU support programs.

Allocation of Funds within SHARE-operations are in 3 sections with corresponding roles:

Function	Owner	Funding source	Description
Survey Operations	Country teams/ National agencies	Member countries + DG EMPL (EUCOV)	Covers data collection, country-specific logistics. SHARE-ERIC acts as intermediary in most cases
Administrative Tasks & Infrastructure	SHARE-ERIC	Participation/ Membership fees	Includes legal, financial admin, software, IT infrastructure (e.g., ~€280 k in 2023)
Scientific & Technical Innovation	SHARE BERLIN + MPISOC (DE)	Project grants (DG RTD, US NIA, etc.)	Supports development of new instruments (e.g., HCAP, biomarkers) and international harmonization

Notably, national funds (from BMBF to SBI in Germany) cover central coordination (~€2.0 M/year), while SHARE-ERIC centralizes much of the budget for harmonization and efficiency

Why the SHARE Business Model Can—And Should—Be Considered for GUIDE

The business model underpinning SHARE is structured around decentralized national financing combined with a centralized coordination system operated by SHARE-ERIC. Each participating country is responsible for covering its national survey operations—typically through ministries, research councils, or national statistical agencies—while the central infrastructure manages harmonization, legal compliance, software development, and scientific innovation. At first glance, GUIDE appears to operate in a different ecosystem. GUIDE has so far depended more heavily on centrally pooled EU funds and top-down governance mechanisms. Although

GUIDE focuses on early-life stages and SHARE on later ones, both are embedded in the life-course approach promoted by the European Research Area and Horizon Europe. In fact, SHARE, Generations and Gender Programme (GGP; Gauthier et al., 2018), ESS, and GUIDE have already engaged in coordinated initiatives such as the SoGreen project (SoGreen, n.d.), jointly proposing integrated approaches to societal transformations including aging, digitalization, and inequality. The challenges facing GUIDE today—financial uncertainty, legal complexity, and infrastructure gaps—are real but not insurmountable. SHARE demonstrates that a decentralized co-financing model is viable even for large, complex, ethically sensitive datasets and offers a practical and proven pathway for building a sustainable, harmonized, and inclusive European child cohort study. Its success across 28 countries in managing a multidisciplinary, ethically sensitive, and resource-intensive infrastructure suggests that, with the right institutional support and political will, the model can indeed be replicated—adjusted, not transplanted—for GUIDE.

Box 10.3: European Social Survey (ESS)

ESS is a research infrastructure that collects comparable data on public attitudes, values, and behaviors across Europe. ESS became an ERIC in 2013 and is led by the Core Scientific Team headquarters at the University of London.

Central Budget for 2023–24: ~€2.95 million

Funding Sources

National contributions from member countries: **~86%**

A total of €2.54 million was contributed by 28 countries. Contributions are weighted according to GDP and population, with key contributors including Germany (€411 k), France (€293 k), the UK (€310 k), and Italy (€219 k).

UK Hosting Fee: **~14%**

As the host of the ESS headquarters, the United Kingdom provides an additional contribution of €408,000, separate from its membership fee.

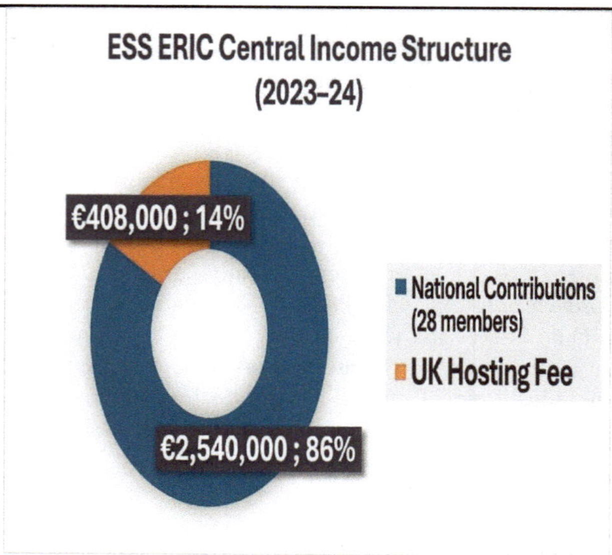

Project-based funding (outside central budget)

The CST also leads and contributes to several major Horizon-funded projects, including:

SUSTAIN-2 (€4.9 M, Horizon 2020)

Infra4NextGen (€9.75 M, Horizon Europe)

ERIC Forum 2, *EOSC Future*, *PAUL*, and *Survey Futures (UK)*

These projects support innovation, digital transformation, and service expansion, but are not included in the core central income reported above.

Outputs: ESS has successfully completed over 500,000 interviews since 2002 and underpins more than 7000 academic publications, highlighting its value as a trusted source of longitudinal and comparative social science data.

Allocation of Funds within ESS: *Core Functional Allocation of ESS Central Resources*

Function	Owner	Funding source	Description
National Data Collection	National Teams (28 countries)	National research budgets	Interviewing, sampling, local logistics, self-completion transition (where piloted)
Central Coordination (CST)	ESS Core Scientific Team (8 orgs)	National contributions + UK fee	Questionnaire design, data processing, survey standards, governance, legal issues
Innovation & Development Projects	CST + Research Partners	Horizon Europe, ESRC, etc.	CRONOS web panel, Infra4NextGen, administrative data linkage, new methods

The ESS Business Model: Possible Implications for GUIDE

The business model developed by ESS combines national co-financing for fieldwork with a centrally coordinated scientific and administrative framework. This hybrid governance model, like that of SHARE, has proven both cost-effective and sustainable over more than two decades and across 30 European countries (see Box 10.3). Despite differences in target populations, both ESS and GUIDE operate in fields that require complex data collection, ethical safeguards, and long-term political commitment.

The experience of ESS illustrates that even methodologically demanding and resource-intensive infrastructures can be maintained through shared public responsibility and targeted innovation funding. GUIDE could adapt this model incrementally, introducing national co-funding mechanisms where possible, supported by EU transition instruments, and building a central coordination body akin to the ESS CST. If successfully implemented, this would represent a decisive step toward long-term institutional stability and scientific impact for GUIDE.

Concluding Remarks

As Europe continues to grapple with complex challenges, ranging from economic inequality to public health crises, investing in research that focuses on child well-being becomes not only a moral imperative but also a strategic necessity. The socioeconomic analysis emphasizes the multifaceted benefits that GUIDE is poised to deliver, from enhancing research efficiency and knowledge output to accumulating human capital and directly benefiting end-users such as children and youth. Financial sustainability is a critical component of GUIDE's potential impact. Financial models of established research infrastructures such as SHARE and ESS offer valuable lessons of diversifying funding sources, fostering cross-national collaborations, and securing long-term commitments. GUIDE's high-quality, longitudinal data will give stakeholders the insights needed to design and implement effective interventions that enhance the lives of children and young people across Europe, creating a more equitable, prosperous, and healthy society for future generations.

References

Agostinelli, F., Doepke, M., Sorrenti, G., & Zilibotti, F. (2022). When the great equalizer shuts down: Schools, peers, and parents in pandemic times. *Journal of Public Economics, 206*, Article 104574. https://doi.org/10.1016/j.jpubeco.2021.104574

Aizer, A., & Currie, J. (2019). Lead and juvenile delinquency: New evidence from linked birth, school, and juvenile detention records. *Review of Economics and Statistics, 101*(4), 575–587.

Almond, D., Currie, J., & Duque, V. (2018). Childhood circumstances and adult outcomes: Act II. *Journal of Economic Literature, 56*(4), 1360–1446. https://doi.org/10.1257/jel.20171164

Attanasio, O., Cattan, S., & Meghir, C. (2022). Early childhood development, human capital, and poverty. *Annual Review of Economics, 14*, 853–892. https://doi.org/10.1146/annurev-economics-092821-053234

Börsch-Supan, A., Axt, K., Beck, P., Bergmann, M., Gruber, S., Máté, V., Oepen, A., Scherpenzeel, A., Schmidutz, D., & Schuller, K. (2019). *SHARE annual activity report 2018/19*. SHARE-ERIC. https://share-eric.eu/fileadmin/user_upload/Other_Publications/Annual_Activity_Reports/SHARE_AnnualActivityReport_2018-19.pdf

Börsch-Supan, A., Axt, K., Beck, P., Bergmann, M., Bristle, J., Börsch-Supan, M., Douhou, S., Gruber, S., Herold, I., Knoblechner, J., Máté, V., Oepen, A., Sand, G., Scherpenzeel, A., Schuller, K., & Weiss, L. (2020). *SHARE annual activity report 2019/20*. Max Planck Institute for Social Law and Social Policy, Munich Center for the Economics of Aging. https://share-eric.eu/fileadmin/user_upload/Other_Publications/Annual_Activity_Reports/SHARE_AnnualActivityReport_2019-2020.pdf

Börsch-Supan, A., Axt, K., Bergmann, M., Bethmann, A., Bristle, J., Börsch-Supan, M., Coscia, V., Douhou, S., Gruber, S., Knoblechner, J., López-Falcón, D. M., Máté, V., Oepen, A., Pettinicchi, Y., Sand, G., Schuller, K., Sommer, E., & Stuck, S. (2021). *SHARE annual activity report 2020/21*. Max Planck Institute for Social Law and Social Policy, Munich Center for the Economics of Aging. https://share-eric.eu/fileadmin/user_upload/Other_Publications/Annual_Activity_Reports/SHARE_AnnualActivityReport2020_WEB.pdf

Börsch-Supan, A., Axt, K., Bergmann, M., Börsch-Supan, M., Coscia, V., Douhou, S., Franzese, F., Gruber, S., Knoblechner, J., Lasson, S., López-Falcón, D. M., Máté, V., Oepen, A., Pettinicchi, Y., Philip, J. T., Sand, G., Schuller, K., Schmidutz, D., Stuck, S., & Yilmaz, A. Y. (2022). *SHARE annual activity report 2021/22*. Max Planck Institute for Social Law and Social Policy, Munich Center for the Economics of Aging. https://share-eric.eu/fileadmin/user_upload/Other_Publications/Annual_Activity_Reports/SHARE-ERIC_AnnualActivityReport2021-22.pdf

Börsch-Supan, A., Axt, K., Becker, S., Bergmann, M., Börsch-Supan, M., Douhou, S., Franzese, F., Gruber, S., Herold, I., Knoblechner, J., Kronschnabl, J., Lasson, S., López-Falcón, D. M., Meinert, F., Pettinicchi, Y., Richter, D., Sand, G., Schuller, K., Stuck, S., Thaler, M., & Uršič, S. (2023). *SHARE annual activity report 2022/23*. Max Planck Institute for Social Law and Social Policy, Munich Center for the Economics of Aging. https://share-eric.eu/fileadmin/user_upload/Other_Publications/Annual_Activity_Reports/SHARE-ERIC_AnnualActivityReport2022-23.pdf

Börsch-Supan, A., Axt, K., Beck, P., Becker, S., Bergmann, M., Börsch-Supan, M., Chłoń-Domińczak, A., Douhou, S., Franzese, F., Gruber, S., Hecher, M., Herold, I., López-Falcón, D. M., Pettinicchi, Y., Richter, D., Sand, G., Schnabel, C., Schuller, K., Schumacher, A., Stuck, S., Thaler, M., Wagner, M., & Yilmaz, A. Y. (2024). *SHARE annual activity report 2023/24*. Max Planck Institute for Social Law and Social Policy, Munich Center for the Economics of Aging. https://share-eric.eu/fileadmin/user_upload/Other_Publications/Annual_Activity_Reports/SHARE-ERIC_AnnualActivityReport2023-24.pdf

Braghieri, L., Levy, R., & Makarin, A. (2022). Social media and mental health. *American Economic Review, 112*(11), 3660–3693. https://doi.org/10.1257/aer.20211218

Bulman, G., & Fairlie, R. W. (2016). Technology and education: Computers, software, and the internet. In *Handbook of the Economics of Education* (Vol. 5, pp. 239–280). Elsevier.

Caritas. (2021). *Rapporto 2021 su povertà ed esclusione sociale*. https://archivio.caritas.it/pls/caritasitaliana/v3_s2ew_consultazione.mostra_pagina?id_pagina=9651

Chetty, R., Hendren, N., Kline, P., & Saez, E. (2014). Where is the land of opportunity? The geography of intergenerational mobility in the United States. *The Quarterly Journal of Economics, 129*(4), 1553–1623. https://doi.org/10.1093/qje/qju022

Conti, G., & Gupta, S. (2024). Early childhood interventions to reduce intergenerational inequality. In E. Kilpi-Jakonen, J. Blanden, J. Erola, & L. Macmillan (Eds.), *Research handbook on intergenerational inequality* (pp. 342–356). Edward Elgar Publishing.

Cristia, J., Ibarrarán, P., Cueto, S., Santiago, A., & Severín, E. (2017). Technology and child development: Evidence from the One Laptop per Child Program. *American Economic Journal: Applied Economics, 9*(3), 295–320. https://doi.org/10.1257/app.20150385

Cunha, F., Heckman, J. J., Lochner, L., & Masterov, D. V. (2006). Interpreting the evidence on life cycle skill formation. In E. A. Hanushek & F. Welch (Eds.), *Handbook of the economics of education* (Vol. 1, pp. 697–812). Elsevier. https://doi.org/10.1016/S1574-0692(06)01016-6

Cunha, F., & Heckman, J. J. (2007). The technology of skill formation. *American Economic Review, 97*(2), 31–47. https://doi.org/10.1257/aer.97.2.31

Currie, J., & Almond, D. (2011). Human capital development before age five. In O. Ashenfelter & D. Card (Eds.), *Handbook of labor economics* (Vol. 4, Part B, pp. 1315–1486). Elsevier. https://doi.org/10.1016/S0169-7218(11)02413-0

Davidov, E., Schmidt, P., & Schwartz, S. H. (2008). Bringing values back in: The adequacy of the European Social Survey to measure values in 20 countries. *Public Opinion Quarterly, 72*(3), 420–445. https://doi.org/10.1093/poq/nfn035

Doyle, O. (2020). The first 2,000 days and child skills. *Journal of Political Economy, 128*(6), 2067–2122. https://doi.org/10.1086/705707

Duncan, G. J., Ziol-Guest, K. M., & Kalil, A. (2010). Early-childhood poverty and adult attainment, behavior, and health. *Child Development, 81*(1), 306–325. https://doi.org/10.1111/j.1467-8624.2009.01396.x

Ecchia, G., O'Leary, C., & Messori, L. (2021). Ex-ante socio-economic impact assessment for a social science research infrastructure: The case of EuroCohort. *Annals of Public and Cooperative Economics, 92*, 531–563. https://doi.org/10.1111/apce.12346

Ecchia, G., Monfardini, C., Policino, L., & Wakefield, M. (2024). *GUIDE Network Development Work Package D8.4: Policy briefings*. COORDINATE Project, The Manchester Metropolitan University. CORDIS project results page for COORDINATE. https://cordis.europa.eu/project/id/101008589/results

ELFE. (2025). *ELFE—Questionnaires and other useful documents*. https://www.elfe-france.fr/en/the-research/access-to-data-and-questionnaires/questionnaires-and-other-useful-documents/

European Commission. (2024). *Commission Recommendation of 23 April 2024 on developing and strengthening integrated child protection systems in the best interests of the child* (C(2024) 2680 final).

Eurostat. (2024). *People at Risk of Poverty or Social Exclusion*. Eurostat (ilc_peps01n). https://ec.europa.eu/eurostat/statisticsexplained/

Felfe, C., & Lalive, R. (2018). Does early child care affect children's development? *Journal of Public Economics, 159*, 33–53. https://doi.org/10.1016/j.jpubeco.2018.01.012

Florio, M. (2019). *Investing in science: Social cost-benefit analysis of research infrastructures*. MIT Press.

Gauthier, A. H., Cabaço, S., & Emery, T. (2018). Generations and Gender Survey study profile. *Longitudinal and Life Course Studies, 9*(4), 456–465. https://doi.org/10.14301/llcs.v9i4.500

Goudeau, S., Sanrey, C., Stanczak, A., Manstead, A., & Darnon, C. (2021). Why lockdown and distance learning during the COVID-19 pandemic are likely to increase the social class achievement gap. *Nature Human Behaviour, 5*(10), 1273–1281. https://doi.org/10.1038/s41562-021-01212-7

ISTAT. (2024). *Annuario statistico italiano 2024. Capitolo 4, Sanità e salute*. https://www.istat.it/storage/ASI/2024/capitoli/C04.pdf

Kiessling, L., & Norris, J. (2020). *The long-run effects of peers on mental health* (MPI Collective Goods Discussion Paper No. 2020/12). Max Planck Institute for Research on Collective Goods. https://www.econstor.eu/bitstream/10419/229998/1/2020-12online.pdf

Malamud, O., & Pop-Eleches, C. (2011). Home computer use and the development of human capital. *Quarterly Journal of Economics, 126*(2), 987–1027. https://doi.org/10.1093/qje/qjr008

Moulin, F., Bailhache, M., Monnier, M., Thierry, X., Vandentorren, S., Côté, S. M., Falissard, B., Simeon, T., Geay, B., Marchand, L., Dufourg, M. N., Ancel, P. Y., Charles, M. A., Rouquette, A., Melchior, M., Galéra, C., & SAPRIS Study Group. (2023). Longitudinal impact of psychosocial status on children's mental health in the context of COVID-19 pandemic restrictions. *European Child & Adolescent Psychiatry, 32*(6), 1073–1082. https://doi.org/10.1007/s00787-022-02010-w

OECD. (2015). Cost-benefit analysis of investment projects. In *Government at a glance 2015*. OECD Publishing. https://www.aranagenzia.it/attachments/article/6641/Government%20at%20a%20Glance%202015_OECD.pdf

OECD. (2019). *Reference framework for assessing the scientific and socio-economic impact of research infrastructures* (OECD Science, Technology and Industry Policy Paper No. 65). OECD Publishing. https://doi.org/10.1787/3ffee43b-en

OECD. (2025). How's life for children in the digital age? *OECD Publishing*. https://doi.org/10.1787/0854b900-en

Quail, A., Williams, J., McCrory, C., Murray, A., & Thornton, M. (2011). *Sample design and response in wave 1 of the infant cohort (at 9 months) of Growing Up in Ireland*. Department of Health and Children.

Richardson, D., Carraro, A., Cebotari, V., & Gromada, A. (2020). *Supporting families and children beyond COVID-19: Social protection in high-income countries* (Innocenti Research Report). UNICEF Office of Research, Innocenti.

SoGreen. (n.d.). *Tracking the social side of the Green Transition in Europe*. Retrieved December 8, 2025, from https://sogreen-project.eu/

Giovanni Righetto (Ph.D.) is a postdoc Research Fellow in the Growing Up in Digital Europe Preparation Phase (GUIDEPREP) team at the Department of Economics of the University of Bologna. His research interests include political economy, the economics of corruption and the economic impact of social norms, with particular reference to gender norms.

Giulio Ecchia (Ph.D.) is a professor of Economics at the University of Bologna, Italy. He is currently leading the UNIBO team in the Growing Up in Digital Europe (GUIDE) project. His research interests include social innovation and social economy, behavioral economics and the economics of regulation.

Enrico Elefante is a public official at the Italian Youth Agency (AIG) since October 2024. He is a former educational consultant, trainer, and senior consultant for the National Youth Agency (ANG). He recently completed a research fellowship at the University of Bologna for the Growing Up in Digital Europe Preparation Phase (GUIDEPREP) project.

Index

L. K. Taylor et al. (eds.), *Growing Up in Digital Europe*, Springer Series on Child and Family Studies, https://doi.org/10.1007/978-3-032-30592-3

FSC
www.fsc.org
MIX
Papier | Fördert
gute Waldnutzung
FSC® C083411

Kolibri 360 GmbH
Ferdinand-Jühlke-Straße 7
99095 Erfurt, Deutschland
produktsicherheit@kolibri360.de